Perineum Power

for Women

Dhyana Bartkow

with Somatic WAve™

ISBN: 9798650930266

Imprint: Independently published

Published November 2020

CONTENTS

ACKNOWLEDGEMENTS

Special acknowledgement and gratitude go to my parents who provided a foundation both in the material and the spiritual worlds for me as a child. Through their love and nurturance they gave me my first feelings of being safe and grounded on the earth while experiencing a yearning for the mystical.

I thank the following teachers who fueled my knowledge and understanding of body, mind and spirit. They came into my life at times when I was either in the pit of physical pain or at the frontier of new horizons of discovery.

Richard Hittleman's *Yoga 28 Day Exercise Plan* (1969) provided an easy to understand, self-help, first introduction to yoga. Swami Vishnu of the Sivananda Institute introduced me to traditional hatha yoga and meditation in a formal setting. Maureen Tribe, Dr. Bruce Carruthers, and B.K.S. Iyengar himself instructed me regarding precise physical alignment through Iyengar Yoga for several years. Donna Farhi contributed by approaching yoga through intrinsic movement patterns, which she had learned from Bonnie Bainbridge Cohen's School for Body-Mind Centering and which were reinforced by the work of Stanley Keleman. Risa Kaparo introduced me to Vanda Scaravelli's "antiforce yoga" and was instrumental in expanding my experience of Somatic Learning and self-sensing in my yoga practice.

Debbie and Carlos Rosas, creators of The Nia Technique, trained me as a black belt teacher of this holistic barefoot fitness practice, which combines dance, martial and healing arts principles, and advocates listening to sensation. They also exposed me to the work of Stanley Keleman, who described human patterns of physical and emotional development in terms of tubes, pouches and diaphragms.

The Washington Psychic Institute, and later Barbara Ann Brennan's school, taught me in-body meditation, psychic reading and the healing of chakras for emotional and spiritual well-being. Master Mantak Chia and Minke de Vos introduced me to the *chi* meridians and the *tan tien* of Traditional Chinese

Medicine, as well as to the in-body meditation and *chi kung* energy practices of Taoist Healing Love. Michael Reed Gach provided further detailed training on chi meridians, the Twelve Meridian Cycle and Five Elements Theory as it relates to acupressure, well-being and healing.

Thomas W. Myers discovered a "new anatomy" to describe the human body and its movement in terms of fascia rather than isolated muscles, and when I noticed that these myofascial continuities paralleled the chi meridians I had been activating in Taoist energy practices, the last piece of the puzzle was added and the Somatic WAve™ system started to reveal itself to me.

I am deeply grateful to my students, who were trusting and enthusiastic participants during the development of this material. I appreciate their courage, willingness and sense of humour.

I thank Michele Lilyanna for her Rebound drawing and timely encouragement in my initial creative stages as well as Cody Chancellor for his sensitive and artful execution of all other illustrations.

I am in awe and gratitude that, under the most unlikely circumstances, the Universe brought me together with the assiduous editorial expertise of Lynne Willard and the design artistry of Kathleen Ennis to benefit from their skill in the creation of this book.

INTRODUCTION

Congratulations! You are about to uncover a great power within you that will not only enhance your physical well-being and enrich your personal growth, but also bolster and balance the female principle on Gaia and contribute to the evolution of human consciousness in general. My intent is to offer you a new form of body awareness and self-sensing that improves your alignment, wellness and sexuality so that you can taste the beauty of life as a woman more fully.

Take your time absorbing each of the six Somatic WAve™ principles that are used in Perineum Power. Resist rushing to the end. The depth to which you go into each principle will augment the volume and height of your WAve™ of pleasure. At first you will gain benefits by moving your body purely physically. However when you learn to engage all of the principles simultaneously, you will be able to split your awareness between sensation and visualization to move and improve yourself with energy while tapping into the primary energy pattern of the Universe.

As a teacher and founder of Inner Moves Wellness Center, whose life's study and work has been in the realm of movement, meditation and bodywork, over the decades I have had three major opportunities (aka injuries) to formulate the theories presented in this book. They led me to create a new movement technique which I called Somatic WAve™.

A larger book on this subject, particularly as it is applied to yoga and the evolution of body-mind-spirit wellness in general, will be published soon. It is called *Surfing the Somatic WAve™ ~ Moving from the Inside Out.* This smaller manual, *Perineum Power for Women*, will introduce you to the core principles of the Somatic WAve™, as the perineum is its main powerhouse and steering mechanism.

Nevertheless, this self-help guide is not meant to be a substitute for medical attention; some types of pelvic floor dysfunction may require medical assessment from a health professional. Please consult a doctor to rule out the possibility of an infection or other underlying medical issue.

This book is a result of my studies with individuals highlighted in the Acknowledgements, my own experiences healing structural and perineum issues, as well as the experiences of students in Somatic WAve™ Yoga classes and Perineum Power workshops. Be prepared to transform your relationship not only with your pelvic floor and sensuality, but also with your feet, skeletal alignment, chi energy system and sense of center. As your body flourishes, so will your state of mind. Get ready to open your awareness to infinite energy and to welcome more self-assurance and joy into your life!

Includes links to free audio classes:

1. Introduction and Somatic Experience of the Core Diaphragms (Yin Lines)

2. Somatic Experience of the Back Line

3. Embodiment of Love and Light Chakra Meditation

1
LATENT POWER

For centuries, people have been looking for the Fountain of Youth.

What if it existed inside of you?

An astonishing yet latent power lies unused in our perineum in the floor of our torso, so distant from what we usually think of as our control centers—our head or heart. These pelvic floor muscles, which automatically accomplish all the sexual, creation and elimination functions of our body, can also be *consciously* articulated:

- to **energize** the entire body
- to create **youthfulness** despite the progression of years
- to reap the **health benefits of primordial energy** without sex
- to increase **sexual pleasure** and orgasmic response
- to facilitate **movement without strain** to joints
- to **float** into a sense of on-going, non-static internal support
- to **physically self-align** the sacroiliac joints, pelvis and lumbar spine
- to lift the entire physical matrix into **a standing wave**

Just as breathing is an autonomic function that can also be done consciously to access greater states of health, energy and spiritual well-being, learning to control our perineum muscles can bring tremendous physical, emotional, energetic and spiritual benefits.

Thirty percent of women experience pelvic floor disorders!

The weakness of the perineum in the pelvic floor also contributes to a disturbing statistic regarding urinary incontinence. In 2002, it was estimated that half of all women in the United States experience urinary incontinence at some point in their life. Occasional leakage is often ignored until this muscle gives way and becomes uncontrollable but, fortunately, the muscle can be retrained. If underlying infections have been medically ruled out, incontinence (both urinary and fecal) may be avoided with increased awareness and exercise to retrain muscle and nerve reflexes. Otherwise, reflexes can be lost if they are not used (Berzuk, 2002).

In recent history, we who are women have been tremendously disempowered in this part of our anatomy around the world:

- by horrific clitoridectomies that sever this beautiful organ, packed with 8,000 nerve endings, which has no other known purpose besides pleasure
- by cultural taboos that shame us and forbid touching or looking at our own perineum
- by physical, sexual and emotional abuse

Many women forsake developing an inner awareness of their perineum and give away its ownership and control to a sexual partner or a medical professional. No wonder it is weak in so many women! No wonder so many are "turned off."

HOPE AND EMPOWERMENT

Nevertheless, it is encouraging to hear of ancient matriarchies and indigenous cultures, such as the culture of the Hawaiian Islands, who honored the female principle:

> Most rituals could only be achieved through her, for the removal of spiritual restrictions and metaphysical barriers was woman's role… All physical and metaphysical philosophy is anchored to woman for she *is* the Mother of Life and Death and the human proxy for the ancestral and elemental female pantheon (Jensen & Jensen, 2005, p. 41).

Rather than turning off our female power, let's turn it on! Our role in creating not only human life but also balance on earth is great and sacred. To do this, we must stop leaking our female power, at every age and stage of life. It is important to be able to contain it and consciously flower our unique female energy and creative potential. Achieving this starts with the freedom and ownership of our powerful sacred gateway and continues to build through its physical, energetic, erotic, emotional and spiritual awakening and strengthening.

My goal through this book is to bring profound healing and delightful flowering *to* your perineum and, *by means of* your perineum, to your whole being:

- to bring awareness and strength to your pelvic floor
- to bring awareness to the connection between these muscles and breathing
- to bring more health to inner organs
- to enroll your perineum to self-align and strengthen your pelvis and lower back
- to dissolve the "private parts" taboo
- to improve sensual and erotic responses through this bodily awareness
- to increase the sacred female vibratory presence on earth
- to show you how to make and use a Perineum Magic Wand of Empowerment

In each chapter we will systematically develop the awareness skills that will help you move toward *your* personal goals. Strengthening physically while connecting with the felt sense of your inner body (*soma*) develops inner strength by deepening your connection with your inner self.

Your inner strength comes from connecting to this true inner self, which is always talking to you subliminally and guiding you into situations that can help you find growth and personal development in your circumstances. Great things can emerge from your challenges. Our job is to learn to sense and listen… and even to ask the right questions.

Do not surrender your power to the things outside of you and self-doubt. Take responsibility for your destiny. Developing the inner strength that you set in motion here physically will help you center, evolve and trust your personal power!

THREE LEVELS OF ENGAGING

Physiology creates psychology. There are three levels at which you can engage in this self-help method. It is not necessary to choose all of them.

LEVEL ONE – PHYSICAL

By simply fashioning and using the Perineum Magic Wand, you will create a tool that:

- will give you direct biofeedback on your inner muscles
- will give you a way to strengthen these muscles where needed
- will provide traction to create space between vertebrae
- can keep your libido* and hormones healthy
- can increase sexual, erotic pleasure
- can be used as a sex toy if you so desire

* Please note that these Perineum Power practices do not have to be sexual *per se*. Some women no longer pay attention to this part of their body due to negative sexual experiences, a hysterectomy, ill health, or because they think they are too old; however, they are suffering from physical conditions that could be alleviated by these exercises. Simply activating these muscles without any sexual connotation, pulling up to the ovaries and womb (whose energy bodies are still present even if physically removed) and then to the kidneys, increases primordial vitality (*jing chi*) and brings the benefits of strengthened hormonal balance. Distressing menopausal symptoms can be relieved, bones fortified, and vigour increased.

I cannot stress this enough. In Taoist trainings I had learned that not all of women's sexual hormones are created by the ovaries. With these practices a woman is able to enter menopause without distressing symptoms; she is able to remain fully vibrant, continuing to receive hormonal benefits without hormone replacement therapy. I had been doing these practices for a couple years for spiritual and emotional reasons when my menses stopped. After six months I went to my doctor because I thought something might be wrong. She explained "Well you know, you are fifty. You're in menopause." I was dumbstruck to be actually experiencing the easy transition that ancient and modern masters spoke of!

These trainings also stressed the importance of maintaining a circulation of energy up to the brain in order to keep it healthy. I remember one of my female students who had been both in my Chakra Enlightenment and Heart Meditation workshops. When the Healing Love series started she dropped out, explaining that she and her husband were in their fifties and weren't interested in sexual energy anymore. Ten years later she was incapacitated with early dementia.

LEVEL TWO – ENERGETIC

> "I don't believe in age.
> I believe in energy."
>
> *Tao Porchon-Lynch*

The above quote is from a fit and beautiful 97-year-old yoga teacher. If you choose to grow bolder instead of older, take these Perineum Power exercises to a chi (energy) as well as a physical level. Continue on to further chapters to learn how to activate the chi meridian pathways that run through your perineum and to apply the principles of the Somatic WAve™. The unimpeded flow of chi meridians to your organs is associated not only with better physical health and an increased energy level but also with a balancing of the emotional state that is associated with each organ. You can magnify physical and psychological results exponentially by focusing energy consciously.

LEVEL THREE – SPIRITUAL

By connecting Perineum Power exercises to the toroidal energy sphere, chakra meditation, or the Universal Tao Healing Love practices, a most profound in-body elevated state can be experienced.

However if you find scientific details to be initially too heady or off-putting, skip ahead to Chapter 12 IDEOKINESIS and use one of the metaphors to have a somatic experience of a WAve™. It may inspire you to take a look at the illustrations of Lines in Chapter 3 so that your experience can be more profound, and to contemplate the illustration of Perineum Sectors in Chapter 10.

2
SOMA

We are able to self-regulate if we can be conscious and sense what we are doing.

If we cannot sense the muscles of our perineum and internal pelvic floor, how can we regulate them? Accumulated stress or physical trauma may have caused a loss of conscious awareness and loss of voluntary control of this musculature and connective tissue.

SENSORIMOTOR AMNESIA

From my experience of teaching Somatic WAve™ Yoga, I have discovered that many women have sensorimotor amnesia in this all-important part of their body. This is the area of the root chakra, which is responsible for our physical strength, primal energy, grounded presence in a body, and will to live. However, in many women, it hangs like a saggy hammock rather than having the tone of a springboard; it leaks and dissipates life force rather than propelling forward into creativity; it sinks into depression rather than rising to new adventures!

Soma is a Greek word that is used to refer to one's own fluid and subjective corporeal self, experiencing and moving physical parts by proprioception, by self-sensing from the inside and by moving as an "I" rather than an "it." This is very different from moving as a body—an object-level experience of being a thing that is moved around from the outside by imitating how the teacher is moving, how the ideal is described in a book or how you moved 10 years ago. Bodies are often ego-driven and injured. Somas explore and heal in the freedom of "infinite time and no ambition" (Scaravelli, 1991, p. 34).

"The soma, being internally perceived, is categorically distinct from the body, not because the subject is different, but because the mode of viewpoint is different" (Hanna, 1979, p. 198).

Consciousness can be expansive. When you shift from a unidirectional focus on your body from the outside of you to a felt-sense of what is happening inside, your conscious awareness can become omni-directional and non-sequential (i.e., everywhere at the same time). Can you focus inward and enjoy the soma consciousness of sensing your genitals and pelvic floor in concert with the rest of you, right now?

Fogel (2010, para. 5 & 6) calls this "body sense" and points out its healing potential:

> Body sense is medicine. It is nature's perfect blend of psyche and soma in which the practice of attention regulation promoted by slow movement practices combines with the body's readiness to direct its resources toward healing... Links between parasympathetic and immune systems are amplified and strengthened via neural circuitry... Moving slowly and with awareness promotes all of these benefits.

Thomas Hanna, the founder of the field of Somatics, first coined the term "sensorimotor amnesia" to describe a disconnection between consciousness and soma. Does your pelvic floor have amnesia? Has it forgotten how to breathe? How to move voluntarily? How to respond to excitation? Has it forgotten its full sense of aliveness?

The muscle fibers of our perineum and inner core are meant to function in a constant state of tone (Keleman, 1985). However, it is difficult to tone these internal muscles if they no longer respond, if we cannot see or feel them and/or if they no longer send sensory information to the brain. According to Hanna (1979), "Humans perceive a sensory impression only of that for which they already have an established motor response" (p. 198). What motor response is accessible in this part of our soma to give us the beginnings of sensory feedback?

A good first step in self-sensing is using the breath. Through use of the Perineum Magic Wand, a woman is able to amplify her awareness of breathing with this all-important muscle. She can begin to perceive internal sensory feedback from this vulnerable, yet powerful, part of her body. She can start initiating a clarity of voluntary internal muscle control and physical well-being.

This has enormous benefits for anyone suffering from a prolapse of the uterus, bladder or colon, from internal complications during childbirth or from the distress of sexual muscle dysfunction and loss of sexual response and pleasure. Regaining somatic perception and activation in this area restores a vast amount of health, sensuality, self-confidence and freedom.

A balance of tone in these internal muscles is also responsible for the fluid functioning of the left and right sacroiliac joints and of the iliopsoas muscles that move the legs. Using the Wand* (*Signifies short form of Perineum Magic Wand) as a somatic internal exerciser also allows a woman to create internal traction to increase space between the lumbar vertebrae and to self-align her pelvis and lumbar spine.

An injury provided me with the opportunity to discover all of this. A few years ago, I was walking in the forest on a well-worn path when suddenly the land gave way under my left foot. My left leg plunged into a hole in the forest floor all the way up to my left hip socket, hitting my pubic bone against a log just below the surface. X-rays showed that the impact had separated the two sides of my pubic bone, separated my left sacroiliac joint and hip socket and pulled a lumbar vertebra forward eight millimetres. With torn cartilage and ligaments, I had no external support to hold my pelvic bones together. Any pressure on my sacrum was intensely painful; I wore baggy clothing around my pelvis and, for five months, I slept sitting up, propped up with pillows.

Fortunately, I had already discovered and developed Somatic WAve™ Yoga. My studies of the chi meridian system, The Universal Tao chi kung, Dr. Myers' "new anatomy," and Somatic Learning with Risa Kaparo had led me to create a new approach to yoga and to movement itself—a new way based on energy flow within connective tissue and which my body felt was evolutionary.

As synchro-destiny would have it, a close friend was in treatment with a physiotherapist for recurrent urinary tract infections. In the process, she learned that she had very little control of her internal musculature and was sent to sessions with a biofeedback machine. She was also told to use an internal exerciser at home called "The Magic Banana." Because of my background in Taoist Healing Love practices, I sensed the opportunity for my own internal healing and was fortunate to buy one of these exercisers before they disappeared from the market. The Magic Banana was my saving grace to begin strengthening my inside to support my outside.

I have since been able to design a tool that anyone can make at home, which I have found to be even more effective for giving very exact sensory feedback from the various internal muscles, for magnifying sensory signals and for improving somatic awareness. I call it the Perineum Magic Wand.

I am saddened to see so many women dependent upon a cane or walker in order to be mobile. The Wand* might have helped them if they had known about this device and possessed a profound desire and determination to heal themselves.

With the Wand* and your somatic awareness, you become both your own teacher and your own student. You learn from yourself by focusing attention on the sensations inside. This is a form of biofeedback: the mind-body skills curve back on themselves and train themselves; your mind trains your brain's neural system to create new motor skills.

Starting with the Taoist Sexual Energy Kung Fu practices I already knew (Chia & Chia, 1986), I further refined my results by focusing on awakening and strengthening the fascia that was *inside* the injured joints of my pelvis, both physically with resistance exercises using the Wand* and energetically with the Twelve Meridian Cycle, which I will teach you later.

I sensed that my left front and left back perineum quadrants could exert little force in the "sprung" state of this part of my body. However, I perceived a minimal sensation in each area, just enough to direct a slight movement and, through this feedback back and forth, I was able to regain function.

By working to strengthen this internal musculature with feedback from the Wand*, I was gradually able to hold myself together internally and to heal. Resisting a pull on one side of the Perineum Magic Wand activates a specific band of connective tissue along with its inherent chi meridian and WAve™ of energy. It feels like you are pulling a kite string that allows that band of muscle and fascia to simultaneously strengthen and elongate with an eccentric contraction. With a rebound of energy, it floats upward and out at the same time as it is being fortified to create internal support.

I also discovered that, once the vaginal and internal muscles were sufficiently strengthened, they could create enough clamping upward on the tool (particularly with the WAve™) that I could give myself traction by pulling the Wand* toward my feet to relieve the compaction of my lumbar vertebrae. The Wand* has since become my go-to instrument for strengthening and mobilizing my inner musculature, and even for self-adjusting my pelvis and low back at times.

This part of my body is a sensitive area that might have atrophied into a frozen state without this invention. A high-speed motorcycle crash in my twenties threw me on the road and severely injured my pelvis, spine, head and arms. It was the first "accident" that set me on this road of discovery in my body. With the forest floor incident, I had just hit another bump, and another advance.

The Wand* also enlivened my sensual nature with its soft, flexible internal probing, which not only awakened internal pleasure and power, but also fueled a sense of aliveness, desire and impetus in all areas of my personal and professional life.

I am a dancer at heart, and I am extremely grateful to be able to dance freely, with all of myself. I still find it miraculous that I am able to do the things I love as a movement teacher, professional dancer and bodyworker, and I believe that it is my due to share this knowledge with the world.

The injuries were an opportunity for me to "get out of my head" and be more in touch with my soma and, through my physical vessel, to blossom more energetically and in my soul. These were external events that could have crippled me. Sometimes we cannot control what happens in our lives. We can only choose our reactions.

I hope my story will inspire you on *your* road of discovery. As you blossom, the landscape around you will change!

3
SOMATIC WAVE™ COMPONENTS

The perineum is the main pump of the Somatic WAve™. It is useful to gain a basic understanding of the mechanics of this evolutionary technique in order to fully activate Perineum Power in your life. A full treatment of this subject, especially as it pertains to movement and the intrinsic creation of yoga poses, is given in my upcoming book, *Surfing the Somatic WAve™ ~ Moving from the Inside Out.*

This new technique of balanced movement and healing was born when I started to recognize and explore the interplay of myofascial (connective tissue) meridians with *chi* (energy) meridians and "anti-gravity," the latter being a concept first brought forth by Vanda Scaravelli in her book, *Awakening the Spine* (1991).

Somatic Learning intensives with Vanda's student Risa Kaparo in Kauai were integral to expanding my somatic awareness and self-sensing. She introduced me to the concepts of soma, differentiation, anti-force, wave and elongation. As a result, I first experienced my skeleton as "free-floating in a sea of soft tissue," a phrase that Kaparo often used in her workshops.

When I began studying *Anatomy Trains* (2001) and the brilliant discoveries that Thomas Myers had made regarding longitudinal fascial continuities through dissection, I recognized that these connective tissue meridians were also housing the chi meridians, which Myers did not note until his second edition in 2009. Nevertheless, his leading-edge "new anatomy" started to awaken in me an awareness of the *distinct* wave that is available in *each* of the twelve lines of connective tissue by engaging their energy pathways.

At the time, I was also facilitating Healing Love Chi Kung workshops, in which the perineum plays a central role. When these diverse influences all met each other in the yoga classes I was teaching, a far-reaching system of movement, energy work and healing emerged, which I called Somatic WAve™.

SIX SOMATIC WAVE™ PRINCIPLES IN PERINEUM POWER

1. OPPOSING FORCE AND REBOUND

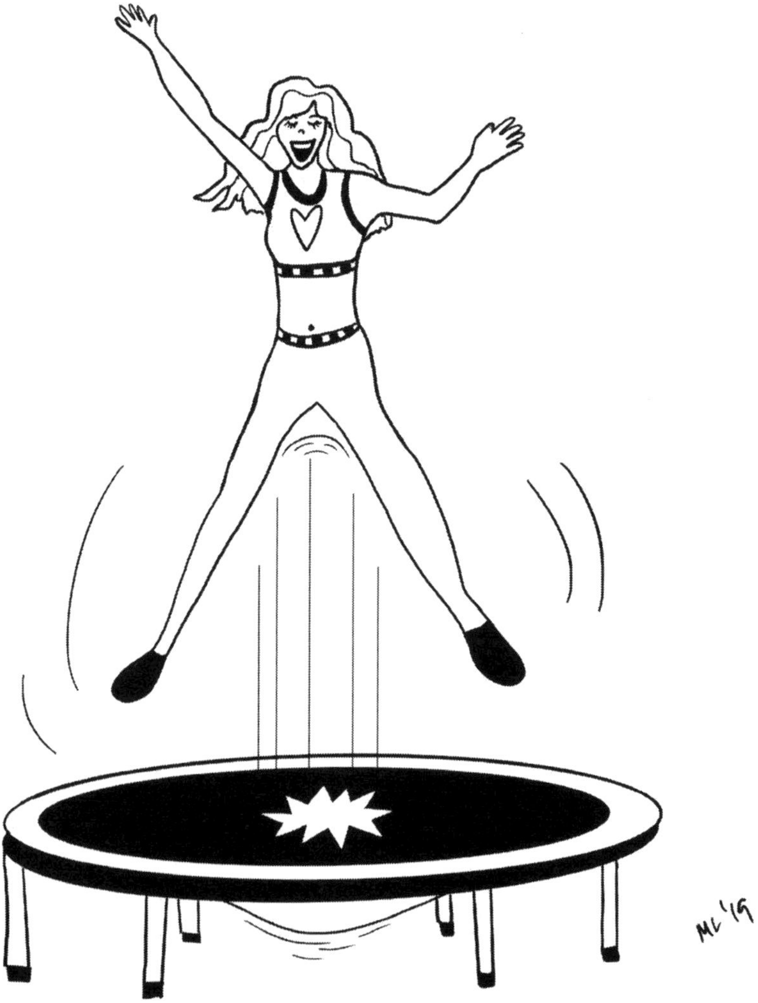

Fig. 1 Rebound

Energy is created at each point where opposing forces:

- touch and propel off each other with a push-away
- or push and pull at the same time

If you try to bring two magnets of the same polarity toward each other, you will feel their Opposing Force and Rebound.

You can create this Rebound:

- by exerting actual physical force against gravity, such as jumping on a trampoline, or by pushing against any immovable object
- as the result of visualization and "felt-sense"

We will do both in Perineum Power.

Newton's third law of motion states that, "For every action there is an equal and opposite reaction." This allows energy to move in a circle. On an esoteric level, it is an element of the mystery of manifestation.

On the human plane, we exist between two strong forces: between the cosmic electromagnetic field that pulls us upward into space and earth gravity that sucks us downward; and between our higher self and our animal self. In this duality, we are constantly either flipping in wide arcs between two opposites or seeking to balance them. In Somatic WAve™, we engage these Opposing Forces simultaneously to create both strength and elongation.

2. YANG-YIN

Yang energy moves downward from the cosmos, and Yin moves upward from the earth along chi meridians that flow through the connective tissue (myofascia) that surrounds our muscles and bones. If you think of energy as a physical reality, it is easier to move with the concept of a continuum that goes down one of your Yang Lines, continues into the earth and Rebounds back up along the corresponding Yin Line.

These Lines are part of a bigger energy system, the toroidal energy sphere that surrounds the earth. You can learn to ride the torus, just like surfers learn to ride an ocean wave that hits the ocean floor as it comes toward shore. The Push-away Point of each Yang Line is the "ocean floor" that determines its Rebound.

The Back Line sends the yang bladder meridian energy over the skull, down the back of the torso and legs along the heel foot and into the earth. Energy then Rebounds from its Push-away Point in gravity up the Deep Core as the yin kidney meridian.

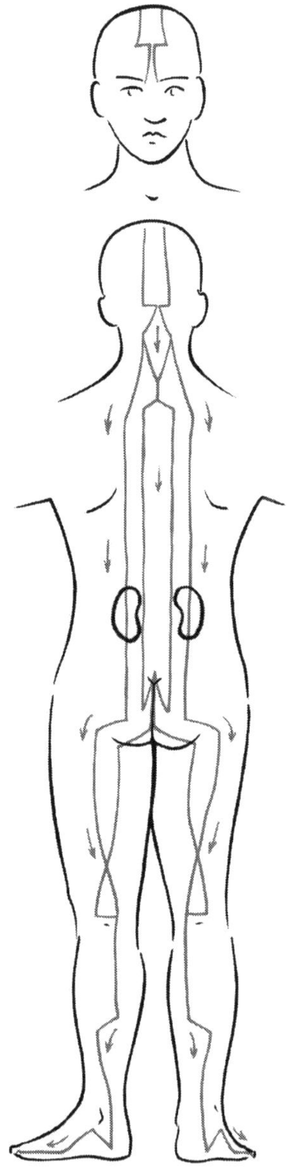

Fig. 2 Yang Bladder
Back Line

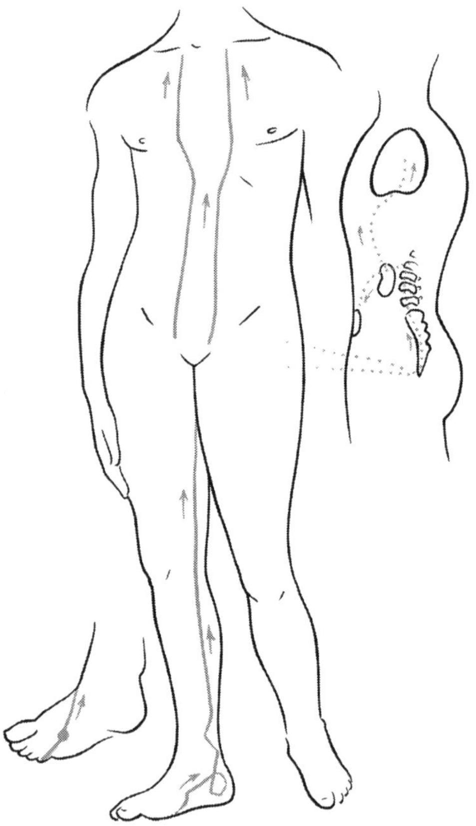

Fig. 3 Yin Kidney
Back Line

"Heel foot" (heel and outer blade of the foot leading to and including 5th and 4th toes) and "toe foot" (bones leading to and including 1st, 2nd and 3rd toes) are anatomical distinctions noted by Ida Rolf, creator of Structural Integration, according to how these bones emanate from the ankle (1987).

The Front Line sends yang stomach meridian energy down the front of the face, torso and legs along the toe foot, and then grounds into the earth through the ball of the foot at the base of the big toe and Rebounds up as the yin spleen meridian.

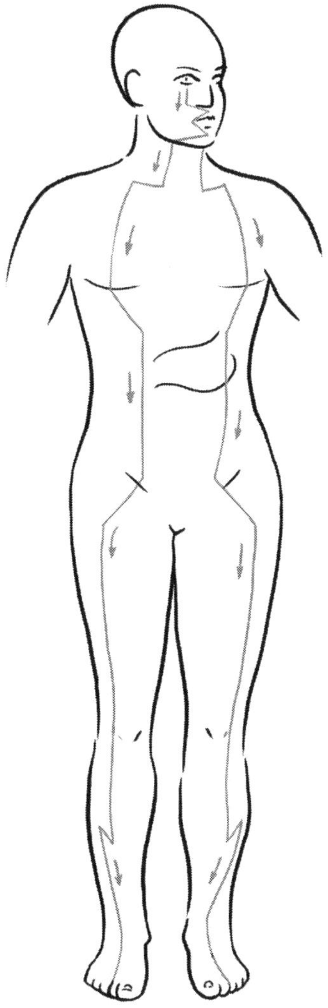

Fig. 4 Yang Stomach
Front Line

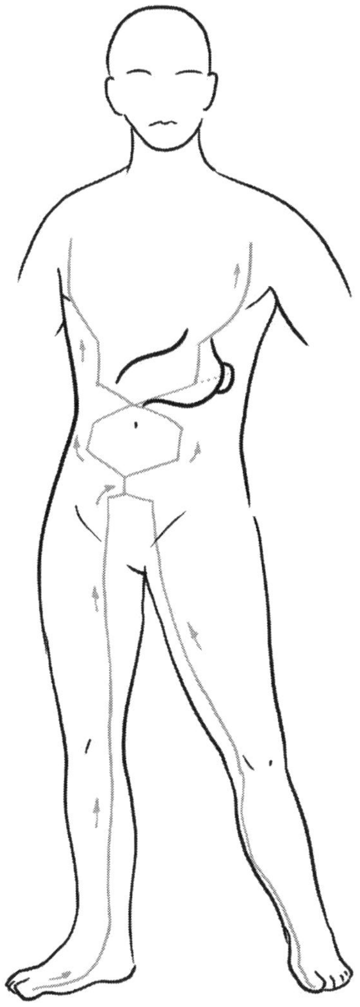

Fig. 5 Yin Spleen
Front Line

The Lateral Line sends yang gall bladder meridian energy along the heel foot, grounding through the metatarsal bone at the base of the 5th toe, and then energy Rebounds up the core from its Push-away Point in the surrounding energy field as the yin liver meridian.

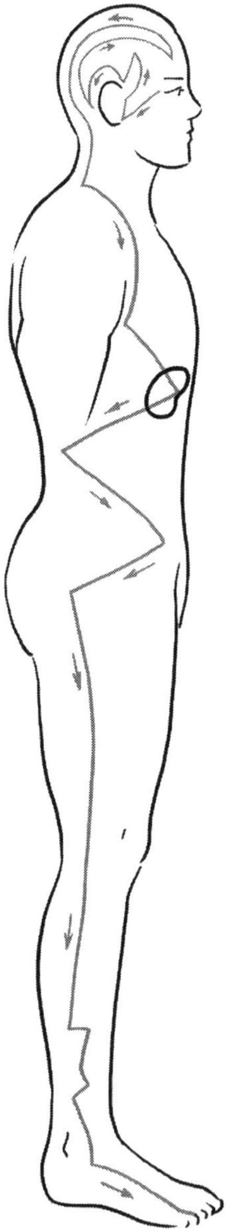

Fig. 6 Yang Gall Bladder Lateral Line

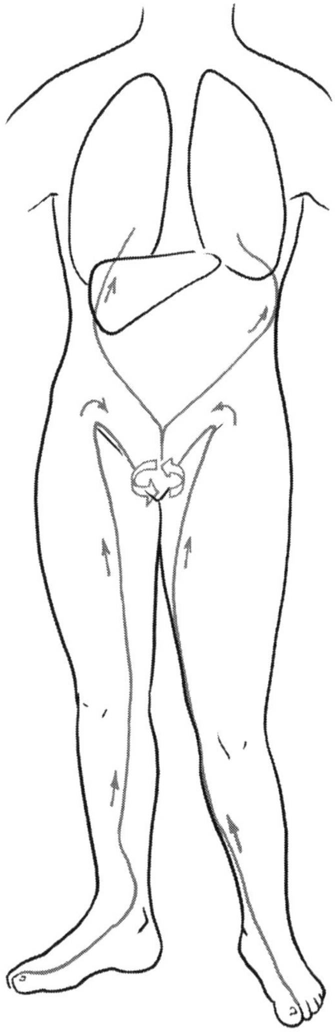

Fig. 7 Yin Liver Lateral Line

3. TENSEGRITY

First coined from the phrase "tension integrity" by Buckminster Fuller, tensegrity is a naturally occurring phenomenon that Fuller recognized and developed with his creation of the geodesic dome. This structure has amazing strength that is self-supported by equalizing tension in all directions. In a tensegrity structure, compression members push out while tension members pull in. If these two forces are balanced, the structure has stability. It also enjoys an equalized state of minimal tension with a maximum amount of strength.

Tensegrity is created within ourselves when we engage Opposing Force to create the omnidirectionality of a Somatic WAve™ moving everywhere at once. When balanced tension is created between the Yang and Yin Lines running through our connective tissue and chi meridians, our bodies develop biotensegrity and become self-supporting, just like a geodesic dome!

I write WAve™ with double capitalization to express this biotensegrity created in our bodies by Opposing Force. The W represents the three Yang Lines descending from the cosmos along our outer body; the A represents the Rebound of Yin Lines pumped up through the inner body along our two legs and two arms by the horizontal diaphragms.

4. PRESS POINTS

These are the points of sensory presence at the bones (feet, tailbone, sit bones, hands), where the meridians extend an energetic vibration into the energy field of the earth or into space to create a Rebounding WAve™ of energy through the entire body. You must extend energy the same distance beyond a Press Point as you want it to Rebound within your soma. In other words, extend energy through a Press Point to a Push-away Point a body length beyond your body if you want to lift and support your *whole* body internally with a Somatic WAve™.

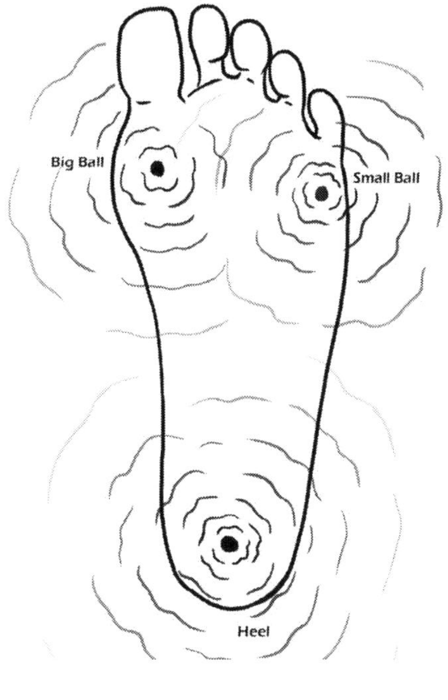

Fig. 8 Feet Press Points

Energy moves in spirals. When the Press Points of the two feet push energy downward while the feet simultaneously try to pull toward each other but can't move, they create an Opposing Force that spirals upward. Magnified by the squeeze inward of the legs, the Rebound moves up into the perineum and ascends the spine like a standing wave.

This helical wind spinner moves in the shape of a standing wave when the wind blows.

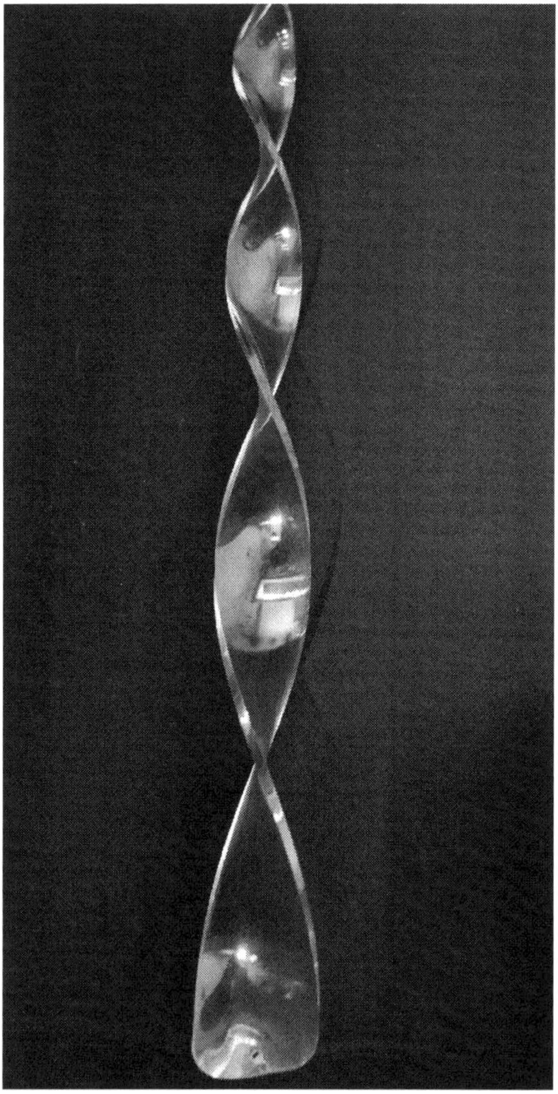

Fig. 9 Standing Wave

5. PERINEUM SECTORS

The main trampoline of your Somatic WAve™ is the perineum. It is the "critical point" where the least effort exerts the greatest effect. The perineum is the diamond-shaped muscular floor at the base of your torso. This muscular diaphragm connects the tailbone of your spine to the sit bones at the back of your pelvic bowl and to the pubic bone at the front of your pelvic bowl.

The perineum is connected to all the other internal diaphragms of your core, and it is able to pump energy, stem cell fluid, cerebrospinal fluid and elongated movement all the way up to your palate and the dural sheath around your brain.

Although this book with its use of the Wand* is specifically tailored toward women, all the six Somatic WAve™ principles outlined here can be used by men to develop self-supporting biotensegrity, systemic health and skeletal alignment.

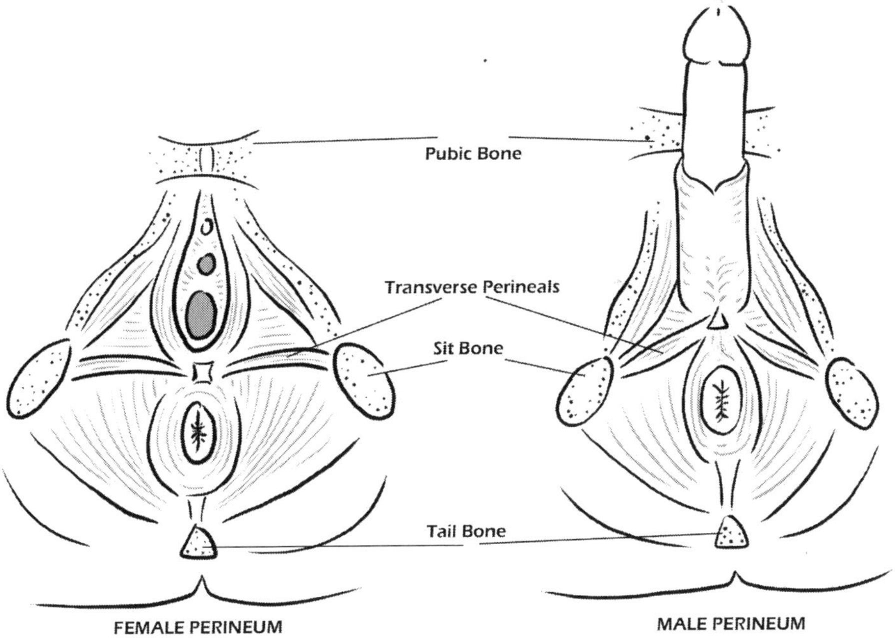

Fig. 10 Female and Male Perineum

Rather than treating it as one sheath moving uniformly, this muscular floor of your pelvis is actually made up of four quadrants and a transverse perineal muscle, each section corresponding to and activating a particular Yin Back, Front or Lateral Line in your Deep Core.

As well as being the main trampoline of the WAve™, your perineum is also the steering house of the WAve™. You can see the major role that the perineum plays in your well-being and why it is important to awaken it to its full potential!

6. IDEOKINESIS

A visualized image can move your soma. Coined from the Greek words *ideo* (thought) and *kinesis* (movement), "ideokinesis is an approach to improving posture, alignment, and fluency of movement through structured guided imagery" (Batson, 2013).

> "The seeing is the doing."
>
> *Krishnamurti*

"Never doubt. It is always possible for the body to carry out whatever has been projected with exactitude by the mind" (Scaravelli, 1991, p. 27).

Simply activating the Yang and Yin Lines of energy, Press Points and Perineum Sectors with ideokinesis creates actual movement of connective tissue and the bones they join! At the onset, you may need to do grosser muscular movements to familiarize yourself with Opposing Force and the ensuing Rebound of the WAve™, but eventually a Rebound can be activated by visualizing energy alone.

By engaging these six principles of the Somatic WAve™, you will find a new key to unlocking ease and natural alignment in your body with the subtlety of attention and visualization.

4
SEXUAL PLEASURE

"Does my sexiness upset you?
Does it come as a surprise that I dance like
I've got diamonds at the meeting of my thighs?"
Maya Angelou

Remember that as a muscle strengthens, it increases in volume and the nerve receptors and reflexes also increase. The common exercise adage, "use it or lose it," refers to sexual muscle function and responsiveness also!

As well as enabling women to consciously articulate, strengthen and energize their entire body, the Perineum Magic Wand can also help them to get in touch with their sexiness and sexual agility. The loop of the Wand* feels surprisingly similar to a human hand or penis in its softness and strength, especially if it is warmed either in water or against the skin before use.

- Women become more orgasmic and deepen their orgasm by strengthening the diamond shape of their perineum and by learning to isolate the components of their internal musculature.

- A healthy muscle is able to relax as well as contract. Similarly, a healthy perineum is able to relax and avoid hypertension, spasm and excessive pain during intercourse.

- The Wand* can also be used during menses to relieve excessive cramping (best used in the shower).

- Women get to know their G-spot. The soft loop at one end of the Wand* can hook around it while the loose ends of the tubing rub and stimulate the clitoris, whose nerves are connected to the G-spot. To locate it, feel for the wrinkly texture of skin on the underside of the "camel hump" of your pubic bone. With stimulation of the clitoris, this area inside the vagina swells and becomes more deliciously sensitive to touch, leading to female ejaculation.

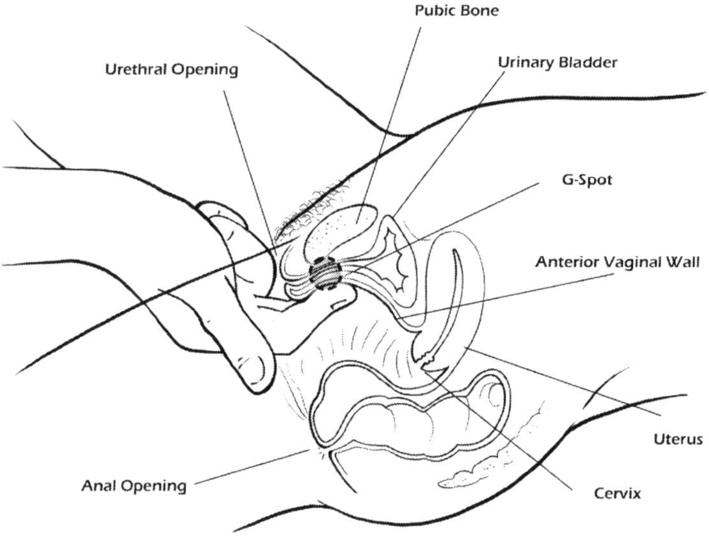

Fig. 11 G-Spot

- Sex and connection with a partner become more satisfying as a woman learns what gives her own self pleasure. She also becomes more self-confident and is able to relax and better tune into her partner.
- All four types of orgasm can be cultivated: clitoral, vaginal, G-spot and cervical.
- The Perineum Magic Wand can even provide a satisfying solo sexual experience. By learning to bring herself to orgasm, a woman's deep tensions can be released and better sleep can be enjoyed.
- The Wand* can also be a tool for spiritual transformation, which will be discussed later.
- It all depends on what our intention is when using it for, as the saying goes: "Sex is all in the head."

The Perineum Magic Wand can be a great tool for transformation on many levels, as it gives us a profound awareness and command of our vital essence.

5
MAKING AND CARE OF YOUR PERINEUM MAGIC WAND

Purchase two feet of surgical latex tubing from a pharmacy. I used tubing that has a ¼" internal diameter and a wall thickness of ⅛", so that the outside diameter is ½". However if that exact size of tubing is not available in your medical supply store, try one that you feel will work for you. There are various diameters and thicknesses available, and it only costs $2.00 to $3.00 CDN per foot, so you can carry out trials if you are not sure how wide or strong your vagina is. Latex-free tubing is available if you have a latex sensitivity. Experiement! I even tried plastic skipping rope at first, although I wouldn't recomend it without knowing what it is made of.

Purchase three feet of plastic-coated clothesline wire at a hardware store, of a diameter that can slide into the interior of the surgical tubing. It will give more resistance to your Wand* for your internal muscles to work against. If you feel that these muscles are weak or you are unsure, do not put the clothesline into the tubing just yet; use the surgical tubing alone at first for the upcoming exercises.

If you wish to provide for more muscle strengthening, slide the clothesline into the surgical tubing so that the two ends stick out an equal distance beyond the tubing. You could also string crystal or stone beads onto the clothesline to fit snuggly against the tubing—beads that are of special significance to you, or whose colors and attributes are related to the chakras and personal qualities you are strengthening. The snug fit of the beads will also help to keep moisture from entering the tubing when washing your Wand*.

Later on, if you have determined that you want the extra stiffness that the clothesline provides, and you have placed your beads, you can assemble the Wand* and dip the ends of the clothesline in glue to coat any rough wire centers and to keep the beads from sliding off.

Leave the Wand* assembled.

Wash after every use.

Store as a loose loop. Either wrap in cloth or sew a fabric bag, using cloth that is aesthetically pleasing to you.

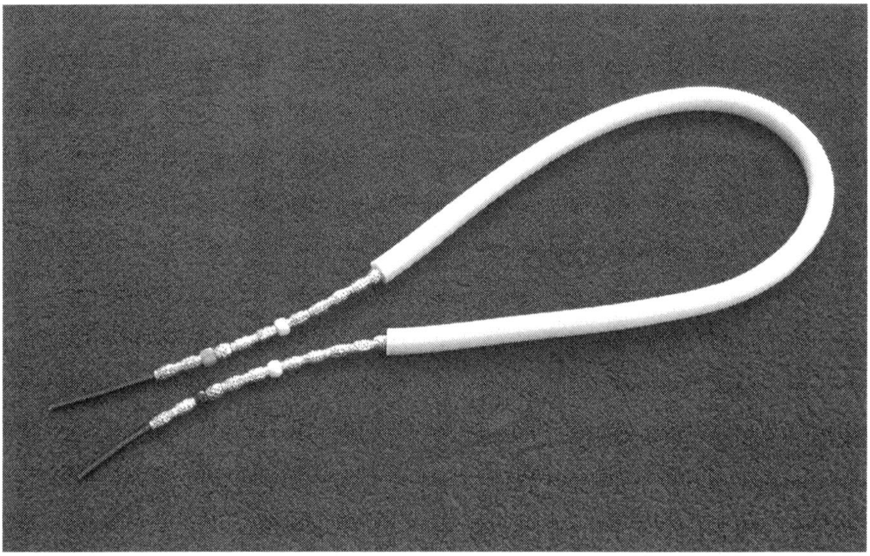

Fig. 12 Perineum Magic Wand

Make this Wand* an instrument of beauty that honours the sacred gateway to your temple.

6
WHAT'S LOVE GOT TO DO WITH IT?

It is important to approach our internal self not only with respect and a sense of infinite time, but especially with love. Our primal sexual energy is then transmuted into a higher frequency that bestows greater life force.

> When we combine our love, compassion and orgasmic sexual energy, a harmonizing resonance arises... our cells will draw in the primordial force and a process of cellular intercourse occurs. DNA is transcribed in the nucleus and translated from RNA in the cytoplasm. Cells divide and combine, giving birth to new and improved cells (Chia, 2016, para. 3).

Ancient Taoists used this activation of sexual energy to strengthen body, mind and spirit. They may not have used the scientific explanation above, but they experienced the results. For thousands of years, sages shared these secret exercises only with the emperors and their concubines, in order to ensure that long life and power be the domain solely of the rulers. Master Mantak Chia dared to bring these techniques to the world during the great unveiling of ancient clandestine practices, which started happening in various cultures in the 1970s. He had to pay many thousands of dollars for these secrets and even mortgaged his house. He was harshly criticized for revealing them globally, but he thought that it was time. I share these details, which he spoke of in his workshops, so that you will know how valuable this information is.

We are extremely fortunate to have the power and longevity of these ancient methods available to us! Yet it requires inspiration and self-discipline to use them, so are they still available only to a chosen few? It is up to you to decide to be one of the chosen.

INNER SMILE HEALING MEDITATION

The following Cosmic Inner Smile (Chia, 2004), adapted from the Universal Tao, will relax your nervous system and create a conducive, stress-free atmosphere, for a deep and peaceful connection with your inner self. It will create the most favourable ground of being for your Perineum Power practice.

As Master Chia and his wife explained (Chia & Chia, 1986, p. 146), "If you have too much negative energy in the organs and do not try to remove it, when you begin to multiply your sexual energy the negative energy will increase, and so will your negative emotions." The following meditation will help to "transform negative emotional energy into good virtue energy."

Sit in a chair with your feet flat on the ground and your eyes closed:

- Imagine the sun shining in front of you and filling your closed eyes with bright light.
- Smile this light out the back of your eyes into the Crystal Room in the center of your head. The Crystal Room is a ball of light about two or three inches in diameter that houses your pituitary and pineal glands, the master glands that regulate all the other glands and hormonal functions of your body.
- Imagine that the light is bouncing off the walls of the Crystal Room, making the light even more dazzling.
- Allow this light also to fill your Crystal Room with the creative love and life force of "the great central sun beyond the sun."
- Smile this light and love from your third eye in the Crystal Room into the thyroid gland in your throat, which controls your metabolism. Feel your thyroid flower open in this light.
- Smile it into the thymus gland behind your breastbone, where your T cells are created. Feel the thymus smile back at you with youthfulness.
- Inhale and bring this inner smile into your lungs, filling every airy pocket with this light and physical sensation of love.
- Smile and inhale it into your heart, so that each beat of your heart pulses light and love through your arteries and throughout your entire vascular system.

- Smile soothing love into your liver and gall bladder, under the right side of your rib cage, thanking them for metabolizing your fats. As you smile, give genuine thanks to the liver for the purification and hundreds of other functions it performs.

- Smile into your pancreas, under the left side of your rib cage, with gratitude for controlling the sugars in your body.

- Smile light and love into your spleen, under the lower left ribs as well. With true appreciation, recognize that your spleen garners energy from your food and breath for the use of the rest of your body.

- Smile love and gratitude into the kidneys, under the bottom and back of your rib cage. Thank your kidneys for purifying your waters and storing your primordial chi. Thank the adrenals on top of the kidneys for their hormonal functions.

- From your kidneys, smile down the ureters into your urinary bladder, appreciating their transportation and holding of these waters.

- Smile into your sexual organs and glands, spiralling them with your love and light. Feel gratitude for their precious gifts of creativity, life force and passion.

- Breathe and draw up their valuable, passionate life force, gushing like a fountain into your tan tien, the energy bank and center of gravity two finger widths below your navel.

- Place your palms on your tan tien and smile into it with gratitude and love.

7
INTENTION AND PREPARATION

Awareness opens consciousness. Intention creates.
Attention energizes.

In a Perineum Power session, your awareness is the catalyst for growth. It can open various fields of consciousness, which can then be directed by your underlying intention and energized by the emotion and frequency of your attention. From sexual release to timeless ecstasy—all is possible as you enter into greater intimacy with yourself and the Universal Field. Just as ancient spiritual texts say that everything in our world is connected, science also asserts that a net or web creates the underlying fabric of all creation. The Universal Field appears to be holographic in nature, in that we are small but perfectly whole pieces of it, able to travel to whatever depths, breadths and heights we intend.

INTENTION

Choose an intention for your perineum session that is personal to you *in each moment*, for example:

"I call forth a union of my body, mind and soul."

"I call forth strength for my inner musculature."

"I call forth health for my inner organs."

"I call forth sensual pleasure."

"I call forth spiritual union."

"I call forth bliss."

EMOTIONAL ENERGY

Awareness simply opens consciousness, but consciousness can vary greatly in its effects, depending upon emotions. Emotions are fields of being that have great power to affect the human brain, energy meridians and organs. Certain fields have higher energy and are greater attractor magnets of health and well-being.

The breakthrough discovery of applied kinesiology in 1971 demonstrated that muscles, organs and acupuncture meridians of the body "instantly went weak in response to unhealthy emotional attitudes or mental stresses" and that this "was accompanied by desynchronization of the cerebral hemispheres" (Hawkins, 2002, p. 61). Through extensive testing of thousands of subjects Hawkins calibrated the relative power of the energy of different feelings, attitudes, world views and spiritual beliefs to promote well-being. On a scale of 1-1,000, shame had the lowest value of 20, guilt 30, fear and anxiety 100; whereas love had a value of 500, bliss 600 and enlightenment between 700 and 1,000.

From these results you can see the importance of releasing any cultural or personal attitudes of shame, guilt or anxiety and instead approaching yourself with healing love in these Perineum Power practices.

Where necessary, be present with the pain of past conditioning and experiences and recognize them as opportunities for growth. Decide to pass through them and release their cellular memory with tears and/or body-work, breathing deeply to bring in more life force in order to heal as you let go of those emotional patterns. As Hawkins says (p. 263) it "requires an extremely focused intent... to escape from the familiar gravity of lower attractor fields and move to the influence of a higher field." Hold to your intention and breathe.

Yoni is a Sanskrit term for the female genitals, a term that naturally imparts a sense of reverence and holiness—of making oneself whole again. A common adage says that the body is the temple of the spirit. Let your yoni be its altar; treat yourself with candlelight baths, rose petals and whatever makes you feel loved and voluptuous as you get to know your yoni in your perineum through this lens of love.

TO BEGIN, HAVE HANDY:

- a tablespoon of coconut oil in a small bowl
- your Perineum Magic Wand
- a washcloth
- a mat or bed to lie down on
- a towel to put under you

GETTING ACQUAINTED WITH YOUR PERINEUM

1. Using a small mirror, look at your perineum. It is the diamond-shaped area of soft tissue that goes from your pubic bone to your left and right sit bones and back to your tailbone. Notice its beautiful resemblance to an orchid. Notice the contours of the muscles that make up this diaphragm.

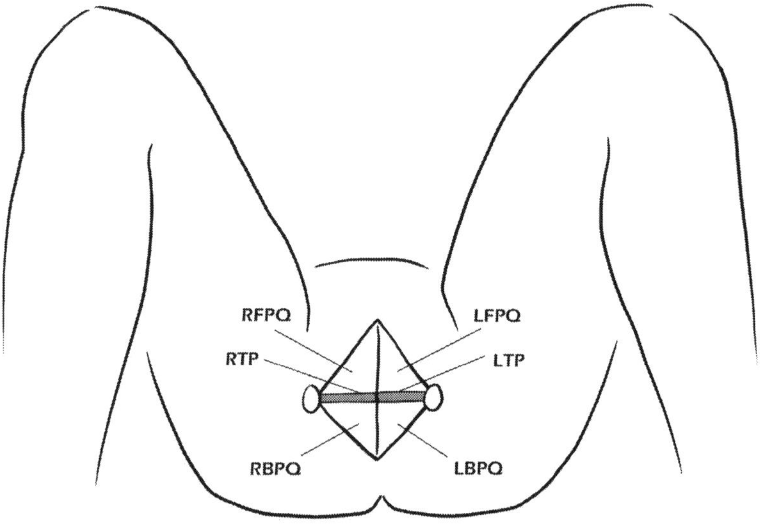

Fig. 13 Perineum Sectors

In Figure 13, RFPQ stands for Right Front Perineum Quadrant, LFPQ stands for Left Front Perineum Quadrant, RTP stands for Right Transverse Perineal, LTP stands for Left Transverse Perineal, RBPQ stands for Right Back Perineum Quadrant, LBPQ stands for Left Back Perineum Quadrant.

Each of the six sectors of the perineum, shown in the diagram above, is a distinct musculature that activates one of the six myofascial and yin chi meridians running throughout your *entire* body! Becoming aware of these differentiations in the perineum is central to the ability to move the muscles of an entire Line consciously and deliver healing energy along it. Can you appreciate the beauty and innate perfection of this resource within you as you explore?

Transverse Perineals:

With oil, massage across the strong muscular band that runs from sit bone to sit bone and divides the perineum into front and back triangles. It is also known as the anatomical perineum.

Front Perineum Triangle:

With oil, massage from the pubic bone at the top of the diamond along its sidewalls to the left and right sit bones. The front perineum triangle moves your vagina. (In males, it moves the testicles.)

Back Perineum Triangle:

Still massaging with oil, follow the sidewalls of the diamond from the left and right sit bones back past your anus to your tailbone at the posterior end of the diamond. The back perineum triangle moves your anus.

Left and Right Differentiation into Six Sectors:

Massage oil along the vertical slit that goes from the center of the anatomical perineum along your vagina up to your clitoris, dividing the front perineum into the muscles of the left front perineum quadrant (LFPQ) and the right front perineum quadrant (RFPQ).

Do the same from the center of the anatomical perineum back through your anus to your tailbone, dividing the back perineum into the muscles of the left back perineum quadrant (LBPQ) and the right back perineum quadrant (RBPQ).

From its center point, the anatomical perineum is divided into the left transverse perineal (LTP) muscle and the right transverse perineal (RTP) muscle.

2. Bend the tubing in half to make a loop and lubricate the loop of the Perineum Magic Wand with coconut oil or saliva.

3. Notice how the elliptical loop takes on a spoon shape. Face the spoon upward toward your pubic bone as you gently and lovingly slip the loop (not the loose ends) into your vagina; doing this will place the loop in the proper position to rub against your G-spot on the internal side of your pubic bone. You may want to explore this area by gently stroking the Wand* back and forth. (If the loop is too big or stiff, remove the clothesline.)

   The G-spot may be a great source of unexplored pleasure for you. It is also the wellspring of female ejaculation. The G-spot swells with fluid upon stimulation, especially if the clitoris—to which it is neurologically connected—is simultaneously massaged between the loose ends of the Wand*.

   The clitoris has a direct relationship to the pineal gland, from which a balancing flow descends to the pituitary, thyroid, thymus, pancreas, adrenals and sex glands (De Vos, 2016).

   You can also increase pleasure and chi flow to your glands and major organs by massaging the breasts and nipples, as they are all connected. The stomach and kidney chi meridians pass through the breasts.

4. Breathe as usual, simply noticing where you feel the Wand*.

5. Go slowly at all times, especially if you feel any discomfort—physical or emotional. Remember your Inner Smile. Stop to rest at any time. When you feel ready, continue to the exercises in the next chapter.

8
BREATHING EXERCISES WITH THE WAND*

Breath is our most precious natural resource —an autonomic function that can also be a conscious bridge into greater health, energy and spiritual well-being.

By increasing your somatic awareness with the following Three Stages of Breathing exercises, you will prepare the appropriate parts of your perineum to be able to coordinate with your breath and feet in the following chapters.

SYNOPSIS

Our breathing patterns of inhale and exhale will follow the progression of a point in sacred geometry:

Stage One	One point is pulsing.
Stage Two	The point becomes a line.
Stage Three	The point becomes omnidirectional and spirals out, similar to the polygonal structure of an acupoint whose top and bottom halves twist in opposite directions when a needle is inserted (Oschman, 2016).

STAGE ONE BREATHING —BEACH BALL BREATH

In the beginning, do this breathing practice *seated* with your feet flat on the floor, *without* leaning back on a chair if possible. This position will train the back of your body to expand and breathe energy as much as the front and sides.

Your lungs are like sponges; they have no muscles of their own and rely on the muscles around them to breathe.

If you have been a chest breather all your life, or if you are constantly compressing your belly in order to appear svelte, you may not feel the Beach Ball Breath expansion of your abdomen because you have become accustomed to using only the muscles between your ribs to breathe instead of your lower thoracic diaphragm.

If this is the case, inhibit your rib movement by placing the palms of your hands firmly on your lower ribs so that they cannot expand when you inhale. Hands inhibiting rib movement will force the thoracic diaphragm under your lungs to expand your abdomen, in order to draw air into your lungs.

STAGE ONE - A: COMPLETE CLEANSING

In order to get in touch with the movement of the perineum, we will start by exploring breath and the diaphragms in general. In the beginning, please engage in this breathing experience without a Wand*.

Belly:

- Full Inhalation: Place your palms below your navel and feel your belly rise up into the warmth of your palms on the inhalation. Feel the spaces between your vertebrae expand in the back of your body. As you draw air in, imagine that your whole torso inflates like a beach ball—from the top of your head to between your legs, everything is inflating and expanding outward.

- Full Exhalation: Squeeze all the air out of your beach ball by contracting your abdominals as well as the diaphragm under your lungs so that the latter moves upward and empties the lungs from below. Allow your pelvis to rock with the breathing. Do not force this movement; only allow it.

Perineum:

- Sit on the edge of the chair so that your perineum is free to move.

- As you inhale, expand the soft tissue between your tailbone, sit bones and pubic bone outward; on the exhale, contract the perineum upward, lifting and supporting your pelvic organs. Ideally the movement of your perineum diaphragm should mirror the upward doming movement of the diaphragm under your lungs when you exhale.

Contracting the perineum upward *with* your abdominals and thoracic diaphragm while exhaling will also retrain the bad habit that people often adopt when exercising or working manually—as they increase intra-abdominal pressure by "pulling their gut in" to support their spine, they often press downward, pushing both the abdominals and the perineum downward, which over-stretches the perineum.

Energy field:

- Energy from the Cosmos: As you inhale, envision your entire body filling with light, as we did during the Inner Smile Meditation. Imagine the pores of your skin—the largest breathing organ of your body—breathing in the life force/prana/chi that is continually showering you from the cosmic field, breathing in photons through your skin and filling the rivers of chi that flow down your body's yang meridians.

- Energy from the Earth: Visualize the moon and silver-blue Earth in space. Just as the moon reflects the light of the sun as a silvery white light, the energy of the Cosmos rebounds from the Earth through us, in the same frequency as our planet Earth—7.83Khz. Imagine that you are breathing in the silver yin energy of our Earth Mother, drawing it upward through the soles of your feet and through your perineum as it expands.

- As you inhale, everything from the top of your head to between your legs is inflating with light from the Cosmos and Earth—expanding outward, upward and downward like a beach ball. As you exhale and squeeze all the air out of your beach ball from above and below, imagine any stale or sickly energy leaving your lungs and the pores of your skin like smoke.

- Continue this cleansing aspect of Stage One Breathing until you feel that you have released all negative physical, emotional and spiritual energy from your body.

STAGE ONE - B: AMASSING CLEAN ENERGY UPON EXHALATION

- Repeat the full inhalation of belly, perineum and energy field with Stage One Breathing.
- Exhale into yourself: As you exhale, squeeze your beach ball by contracting the diaphragms as described above. Squeeze all the air out and visualize that, having released all your energetic debris, your exhale is now able to store the pure inhaled chi as a light in the tan tien of your abdomen. The tan tien (called *hara* in Japanese and The One Point in English) is the sea of energy where chi meridians store energy and from which they can draw.
- Squeeze upward with the pelvic floor, inward with the abdominals and downward with the thoracic diaphragm on top of your lungs, in order to compress this vastness of chi and store it in your tan tien energy bank.
- Located two finger widths below your navel, the tan tien is the central energy hub where the original cell of your conception started to multiply to create all your limbs, spine and organs. All connective tissue radiates from here, and chi meridians flow through this hub, making it our center of gravity and balance. Fill this energy bank as you breathe, and visualize it becoming a ball of light.

STAGE ONE BREATHING LYING DOWN

Now that you have experienced the actions involved in Stage One Breathing while sitting upright, you are ready to do The Beach Ball Breath lying on your back with your knees bent (pillows under your knees if that helps you relax) and feet placed flat on the floor hip-width apart. This position will help you bypass the challenges of gravity on your pelvic floor when we progress to Stages Two and Three Breathing. However, remember to let the back of your body continue to rock, expand physically and breathe energy, even while lying down.

Although the following exercises mainly describe the anatomical aspects of your perineum as it relates to your soma, please remember to approach yourself on a deeper emotional level with respect, love and tenderness as well.

Explore your perineum with breath:

- First place your hands on the bony periphery of your perineum. Prop your head and shoulders up on pillows if necessary, so that your hands can reach down. Place your longest finger on each sit bone and the heel of the thumbs on the pubic bone to form a V so that you can feel the expansion and contraction of your perineum as you breathe.
- Next, slowly insert your lubricated Perineum Magic Wand during an inhalation so that you can start adding sensory feedback from your Wand*.
- Holding the exhale, squeeze a few seconds before relaxing, as if hugging the Wand*. Can you hug equally with the left and right sides of your yoni? Imagine that the light is building inside of you.
- Keep repeating the slow inhale-exhale pulsations mindfully until they feel full, fluid and agile. These pulsations are similar to but more far-reaching and deep-seated than Kegel exercises.
- Now that you feel comfortable with the details involved in diaphragmatic breathing, let your mind rest. Drop fully into your somatic sensing body. Perhaps adding music will help you to let go and access a deeper, soulful layer of self. Feel your whole body expand, receive and embody the sparkle of universal life force as you breathe.

This breathing and strengthening exercise may be enough for your first experience with your perineum and Wand*. Start off slowly and allow your strength and endurance to build gradually.

However, if you continue to the exercises below, keep your Wand* inside. Engage in Stage One Breathing A and B as a resting place for replenishment, and use Stage One as a reference point between all the following yoni practices. It is important to relax, replenish and tune in to how you feel after each one of the exercises.

Also, be mindful that, if you have a sexual partner, your pelvic floor muscles may be tired after sharing intimacy. Give them time to rest and recuperate after sex as well, before exercising with the Wand*, to increase their strength, endurance and agility.

STAGE TWO BREATHING —RAISE YOUR PELVIC FLOOR THREE STORIES

The following is an adaptation of an exercise taught by physiotherapists to treat urinary incontinence (Berzuk, 2002). It strengthens the O-ring muscle which surrounds the urethra as well as the O-ring muscle of the vagina. I experienced a version of this exercise using a jade egg at Healing Love workshops with Taoist instructor Minke De Vos (2016). Although the jade egg has an ancient mystique and vibrational quality, I find that, for these purposes, the springy softness of the Wand* provides a more precise differentiation of the Perineum Sectors, as well as a greater sensitivity to the G-spot.

- Lie down on your back with your feet flat on the floor as close to your sit bones as is comfortable.
- Inhale while inserting your Wand*.
- As you exhale, squeeze inward and upward with your vaginal muscles in three successive stages, like an elevator going from the basement to the upper floors—the main floor is near the opening of your yoni; the second floor is in the middle; the third floor is the uppermost region at your cervix. Hum three rising tones, one at each level. Slowly reverse the process, returning from the third floor to the main floor, which is more difficult. To make this exercise more fun and a part of your life, you may want to put on some music and hum with it!
- Next, go to the basement, as you would to empty your bladder and bowels into the toilet, without straining.
- Your perineum should not be left in the basement! As you go about your daily activities, always maintain a slight tone at the main floor. Return your pelvic floor to a relaxed upward tone after all these exercises, as well as after voiding.

At first, couple the squeezing hug inward with the exhale, and on the inhale feel everything expand outward as you receive more life force through the breath. When you become more practiced, you will be able to move these muscles without association to your breathing cycle. You will also always be able to maintain some tone, even on the inhale, so that your pelvic floor is never loosely hanging like a hammock; instead, it is in a relaxed and easy upward draw.

STAGE THREE BREATHING —REBOUND

Can you feel the left and right sides of your vagina contracting equally against the Wand*?

- To bring more felt sense awareness to the left side of your perineum, gently pull outward on the left loose end of the Wand*.
- Simultaneously exhale and resist the pull outward by contracting the left side of your yoni against the Wand*, in order to pull inward and upward to the third floor. This action creates Opposing Force and a Rebound, like pulling on a kite string so the kite goes higher, or like a horse pulling against the reins to go its own way, challenging you to take more control of the reins in your perineum by pulling inward, upward and bucking! Yippee Ka Yay! Rebound is the beginning of omnidirectional movement.
- Do the same with the right side, pulling outward on the loose right side of the Wand*, as you pull inward and upward with the right side of your vagina.
- Return to the Beach Ball Breath to replenish.
- Take a break. Remove your Perineum Magic Wand and rest. Breathe. Sense. Make good friends with this part of your body.

Notice if one side felt more sluggish and unable to expand or contract. In the future, work more on the side that is listless and underactive, using biofeedback from the Wand*. Focus on the lethargic side to distinguish further whether it is the front, lateral or posterior portion that has amnesia.

This is the beginning of Stage Three Breathing, in which the exhale creates a Rebound and an omnidirectional WAve™ of energy through your core. This Somatic WAve™ will deepen when you add your feet to the process in the following chapter.

But first, please take time repeating the steps in this chapter as much as you need to in order to develop the somatic awareness, movement and strength of your perineum musculature. This is your main pump, powerhouse and steering mechanism. Give it all the time it needs to recover from sensorimotor amnesia as you augment its cellular memory.

Continue to bring more awareness to your breath in general throughout your day.

> "Breathe as deeply as you want to heal."
>
> *Michael Reed Gach*

9
AWARENESS OF FEET PRESS POINTS

"The human foot is a masterpiece of engineering and a work of art."

Leonardo da Vinci

In Chapter 1, it was pointed out that you can take Perineum Power to many levels. Using the information in the first eight chapters, you have enough guidance to strengthen your perineum, support your pelvic organs and improve your sexual response on a purely physical level.

If you wish to start expanding your perineum practice to an energetic level by adding more precise use of your chi meridian system, please follow along. An added benefit is that these exercises will also enable you to correct physical alignment issues in your feet.

Our feet ground the energy that is continually flowing upon us from above (like lightning rods ground electricity) and they can guide the earth energy they contact back up into our bodies.

Creating an aligned connection to earth energy through the feet is important for two reasons:

1. The piezoelectric magnetic force from the earth grows our bones according to how our feet are placed. You have probably heard that weight-bearing exercise is recommended to prevent osteoporosis. This is because the plate-like structure toward the center of our bones grows and contours them in response to how the compression forces of our weight meet the earth. If your feet meet the earth in an aligned manner as you

walk, your feet roll from heel to toe along a central gait line; not doing this results in a walk with most of your weight on the outside or inside of your feet, and you are likely to develop problems and pain in the structure of your knees and hips.

2. In order to create alignment you must beceome aware of the Press Points in your feet. A Press Point of a foot is one of the three *precise* points on the bottom of the foot through which an energetic extension of a Yang Line is sent to a Push-away Point, either in the earth or in the space around you.

The Push-away Point is like a trampoline in the energy field. It creates a Rebound of the yang energy into the reciprocal Yin Line of your inner core. In order for the WAve™ to Rebound up your core and support your entire body, the Push-away Point must be at least a body length away from your Press Point and you must maintain partial attention there.

By learning to activate the three yang Press Points of each foot in this chapter, you will be able to steer energy into a specific yin meridian. This energy will be magnified and pumped throughout your entire body by the corresponding sector of your perineum to create:

- increased health of your organs and glands
- spacious decompression of joints
- eccentric strengthening of muscles
- self-supporting equipoise
- alignment of bones

A TRIANGLE OF SUPPORT

The visionary architect Buckminster Fuller believed that the most stable geometric shape is the triangle. Look at the soles of your feet. Notice the triangle of support in your feet and on the diagram below. The importance of these three Press Points is highlighted by the fact that they are in the most prominent bones on the soles of your feet, which have grown that way to support the human body's verticality.

Each of these three Press Points is *in the center of* a large bone at the bottom of a Yang Line of fascia, through whose yang chi meridian you can send cosmic energy down into the earth like a root.

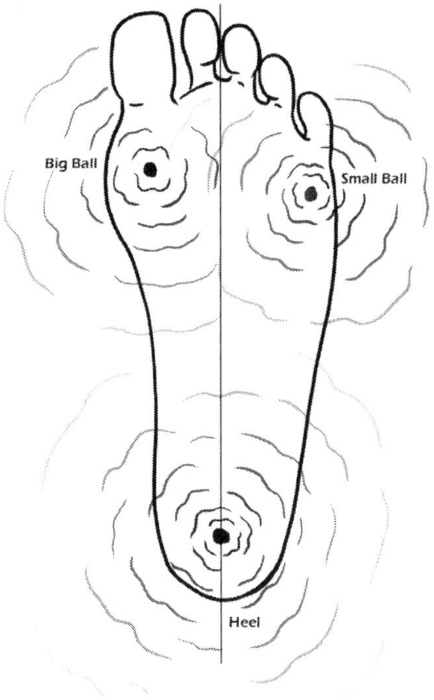

Fig. 14 Foot Press Points with Gait Line

Remember that fascia is a longitudinal continuity of connective tissue, similar to a sausage casing, which surrounds and permeates a grouping of muscles and bones from head to foot, as well as housing a chi meridian (Myers, 2009). If the root descends far enough, it can energetically support the whole height of your body above ground. Yin earth energy will then Rebound from the earth up an adjacent part of your foot to activate the yin meridian that carries potent chi and stem cell fluid to your inner organs.

A consolidation of all the details that are involved when working with the Back, Front and Lateral Lines will be given in Chapters 14, 15, 16. Start to build your sensory awareness and understanding of the role that your feet have on these Lines.

Heel Press Points

The left and right Heels are located *in the center of* the heel bones. (Please note that when I capitalize "Heel," I am referring to the Press Point rather than the anatomical heel.) They are the Press Points of the left and right foot's Yang Back Line, the connective tissue that houses a yang bladder meridian on each side of your outer back body, from your head to your foot. The Heel extends Yang Back Line energy into the earth, which then Rebounds back up in the connective tissue of its reciprocal Yin Back Line as the yin kidney meridian of the inner body, which then flows into the yin pericardium meridian in the chest.

Big Ball Press Points

The left and right Big Balls are located *in the center of* the metatarsal ball of the foot at the base of the big toe. They are the Press Points of the left and right foot's Yang Front Line, the connective tissue continuities that house a yang stomach meridian on each side of your outer front body, from your face to your foot. The Big Ball roots the Yang Front Line further, and energy then

Rebounds from gravity up the connective tissue of the corresponding Yin Front Line in your core as the yin spleen meridian of your inner body, which then joins into the yin heart meridian.

Small Ball Press Points

The left and right Small Balls are located *in the center of* the metatarsal ball of the foot at the base of the 5th toe. They are the Press Points of the left and right foot's Yang Lateral Line, the myofascial continuities on the outer body that house a yang gall bladder meridian down each lateral side from head to foot. The Small Ball roots energy further into the earth and then Rebounds into the foot and up the core as the yin liver meridian of the Yin Lateral Line, which then continues to flow into the yin lung meridian on that side of your inner body.

HEALING YOUR FEET

With this knowledge you will also be able to heal the problems that mis-alignment has created in your feet and consequently throughout your entire frame. These could have started due to injuries, constraining and improper footwear, or due to emotional and physical patterns that were mimicked from your family while growing up.

The earliest photos that I see of myself as a child show fallen arches. Despite orthotics at various stages of my life, my arches never corrected and this translated to a slackness of the connected Yin Lines. Can you feel how it changes your ground of being when your arches lift and a feeling of greater presence and self-confidence rises up and lifts your inner core? Physiology and psychology are deeply connected.

Over a period of time working with the Press Points and Somatic WAve™ I was able to exercise and correct my left foot. Keeping the centers of the Heel and Small Ball grounded while I articulated the Big Ball to lower it precisely, I lifted and strengthened my arch muscles and created a natural shift in the bones of the arch that was reinforced by the rebounding WAve™; the bony lump that I had felt where the tuberosity of the metatarsal joined the cuneiform bone retracted into my foot. However the realignment was hampered in my right foot by an old impact injury that had left bone chips and osteophytes on the top of my foot; they were fusing my big toe and 2nd toe metatarsals together and creating a block sensation that hampered the necessary interplay of all twenty seven bones of my foot.

When I had these osteophytes removed surgically I was able to work with the Big Ball Press Point and start to strengthen the muscles in the medial arch. However the weeks of immobility wearing an AirCast Boot left the bottom of my foot sore to step on and swelling quickly whenever it was lowered for any length of time… until I was able to get down on the floor again to do a Lying Twist with Somatic WAve™. I sent a WAve™ down the Lateral Line to the Small Ball and felt a clicking go through the bones on the lateral side of my foot as it reached that Press Point. My foot realigned on the Rebound. The swelling went away immediately and I was able to walk on it comfortably again.

STAGE TWO BREATHING DEEPENED

EXHALE THROUGH FEET PRESS POINTS

In order to create a more powerful connection to feet Press Points, we will further develop the Stage Two Breathing that was introduced in an earlier chapter. As always, begin with a complete Beach Ball Breath to accumulate energy. As you continue to a Stage Two exhale, squeeze the abdominal diaphragms inward and upward against the sea of energy in your lower tan tien. Imagine and sense that pressure against this storehouse of chi releases an increased flow down the Yang Front, Back and Lateral Lines of your hips and legs, through their feet Press Points deep into the earth.

PRESS POINT AWARENESS AND FOOT STRENGTHENING, SEATED

This initial series of foot strengthening exercises will be done *without the Wand** while seated on a chair. Keep your feet in your awareness and repeat these exercises throughout the day whenever you can.

Massage the bottom of each foot and put your fingers in the soft area between the Press Points. Try to grasp your fingers with your feet to get a sense of the muscles that create the arches of your feet. Imagine that this grasping action of your three arches is sucking your fingers up into your leg.

Sit with your sit bones on the edge of the chair so that your perineum is free to move rather than compressed against the chair bottom. Place your bare feet flat on the floor, hip socket-width apart. Feel the contact of the three Press Points of each foot with the floor. We will start with the Heel, as it has the biggest bone and, therefore, is the most prominent in our sensory awareness.

Heel Press Points:

- Inhale and lift one Heel, without losing contact with the other two Press Points of this foot.

- With a Stage Two exhale as described above, slowly squish this Heel Press Point down, right through the center of the heel bone as if you were trying to squish a small grape deep into the earth. Notice what has to shift in the inner or outer side of your foot in order to bring contact to the very center of the heel bone.

- Still maintaining contact with the centers of the other two Press Points, alternately squish the left and right Heels slowly, simultaneously lengthening out through the 5th toe at the end of the Bladder meridian. Send roots at least a body length into the earth, until both Heels feel deeply rooted.

Notice the grounding sensation going down the entire back of your body. Keep your joints soft all the way down each myofascial continuity, rather than locking them. As you feel a Heel root a body length to its Push-away Point, can you also feel a Rebound of energy ascending the sole of your foot? In chi kung, this area in the central arch is called Bubbling Springs. The Rebound will open the back of your knee, hip and sacrum if your joints remain soft. Eventually you may become aware of it moving all the way up your spine, creating space and floating the back of your neck and head up.

Big Ball Press Points:

- Keep the Heel, *in the very center* of the heel bone, continually rooted as we progress to the next biggest Press Point. Be aware that it is going to try to shift slightly!

- Keep all toe tips on the ground. As you inhale, lift the Big Ball (but not the big toe) and on the exhale press it into the ground a body length, simultaneously lengthening out through the 2nd toe, which is the end of the Stomach meridian. Feel the medial arch strengthen along the inner side of your foot and naturally lift the arch as it strengthens.

- As the Big Ball roots a body length to its Push-away Point with soft joints, can you also feel a Rebound of energy lifting the medial arch of your inner foot and ascending up your inner leg?

Practice this sequence one foot at a time until you can keep the Big Ball Press Point, *in the very center* of that metatarsal bone, rooted deeply along with the Heel, and then go on to the other foot. Notice the sensation grounding down the front of your body into the earth. Keep your joints soft. You may feel a shift in the alignment of your inner knee, as well as the need to turn your thighbone in your hip socket, in order to accommodate the positioning and grounding of these Press Points. This Rebound will strengthen the inner knee ligaments and create space in the knee, front hip socket and groin. It is an excellent exercise to counter knee and hip pain. Eventually you may feel it lift your breast bone and upper palate, so that your shoulder blades naturally relax and slide down your back like the other end of a teeter totter.

Small Ball Press Points:

- Keeping all toe tips on the ground and the Heel and Big Ball rooted as you inhale, lift the Small Ball (this may just be a hair's breadth); on the exhale, root it deeply into the ground, simultaneously lengthening out through the 4th toe at the end of the Gall Bladder meridian. Feel the transverse arch between the Big Ball and Small Ball lifting and strengthening.

- As the Small Ball Press Point descends energy a body length, keep your joints soft. Can you also feel a Rebound of energy from its Push-away Point ascending the lateral side of your leg into your outer hip?

Practice this sequence one foot at a time until you can keep its Small Ball rooted, and then go on to the other foot. Notice the sensation going down the right and left lateral sides of your body. This Rebound will strengthen the outer knee ligaments, create space in your knee and decompress your outer hip socket. Eventually you may become aware of it moving all the way up the side of you body to release your jaw and ear canals.

To Intensify Arch Strengthening and Rebound with Opposing Force:

- Place a very thick, stiff elastic band around your big toes, stretching it so that you once more place your feet a few inches apart. Repeat the seated foot exercises with this added resistance when you are ready to intensify strengthening.

- Ground directly through the Big Balls into the earth to resist the pull of the elastic.

- Feel the amplified working of the medial and transverse arches of your feet.
- Feel an increase in the energy lift that emanates from these arches all along the calves, knees and thighs.
- You may even start to feel the energy move into your perineum. The next chapter will elucidate the connection between the arches of your feet and the perineum.

To increase this lift, increase the Opposing Force by squeezing a yoga block or book between your shins while doing the above steps; squeeze the block between your knees; squeeze it between your inner thighs. Imagine that you are a whale, with feet joined together in a single flipper and inner legs joined by the yoga block into a united sensation of whale tail undulating up and down on an ocean wave as you push off against the floor. By adding the Opposing Force of an inner squeeze to the downward pressure of the Press Points, you will increase the Rebound that strengthens your arches, knees and groins and opens your hips.

STAGE THREE BREATHING DEEPENED

USE IMAGINATION AND IDEOKINESIS

- Stand up (still without the Wand*).
- Bring your feet together and send all six Press Points deep into the earth on an exhale.
- Imagine that you are breaking through to a geyser.
- Imagine the water gushing up Bubbling Springs, along your inner arches, ankles, shins, knees and thighs, and then sucked up into your Perineum Sectors as you push down with your feet.

You may feel how just the slightest pressure on one of the Press Points will create a standing WAve™ throughout your body. This is the beginning of Stage Three Breathing, with which you are able to create conscious movement of a Somatic WAve™ by activating specific areas of your feet and perineum simultaneously.

FEET AND PERINEUM ACTIVATION WITH WAND*

Having worked systematically, training yourself through various steps to have greater sensory presence in new parts of your body, you are now near the culmination of your efforts.

Press Point Down! Perineum Up!

- Lie on your back on a mat, feet placed hip-width apart as close to your sit bones as is comfortable.
- In this reclining position, repeat the same sequence of Stage Two foot strengthening exercises at each Press Point that you did while seated and without your Wand* initially.
- Rest and replenish before continuing.
- Inhale while consciously and lovingly inserting the Perineum Magic Wand.
- Repeat all the exercises once more, but now add Opposing Force on the Wand*. As you exhale and ground down through a foot Press Point, pull the Wand* outward with one hand, and resist the pull by drawing your perineum inward and upward.

This is a close replication of the muscular and energetic activations that can be applied to enhance sexual pleasure, whether with a partner or with yourself. You will find that the addition of foot grounding greatly enhances the Rebound, which in this instance can be an orgasm, rising as high in your soma as your feet root down while the perineum is squeezing inward and upward.

Can you sense which section of your perineum creates the strongest pull upward on the Wand*, as well as which Press Point presses down concurrently, to create the greatest Rebound and floating WAve™ up into your body? The following chapter will give you more guidance and opportunities to explore the six sectors of your perineum with a Wand*.

But first, practice this association of your breath, Press Points and perineum without the Wand* at random moments throughout the day. You will start to feel a physical integration of your soma that will lead to a deeper awareness of the signals communicated to you by the interrelatedness of all your subtle bodies—somatic, emotional, mental and spiritual.

For me, Somatic WAve™ was a chanelled experience first, a synthesis drawn subconsciously, or perhaps superconsciously, from various influences and studies, at times when I needed healing. I am grateful that it is possible to analyse, outline and communicate its components so that it can also be experienced somatically by others. I believe it to be an evolutionary technqiue with many applications and ramifications. Although the analysis and practice of the WAve™ in a point-form, left-brain manner may be methodical initially, eventually you will be able to reap the benefits and embody it easily with the wonderfully soft and profound proficiency of your felt-senses, in whatever circumstance and application you choose.

10
AWARENESS AND STRENGTHENING OF PERINEUM SECTORS

It is possible to simply push physically or energetically down a Yang Line into the energy field and get a slight bounce back. However if you create a Somatic WAve™ that also engages the feet and perineum precisely, there is a fullness to the Rebound that is augmented in all of the energy and physical body. It spreads from the inside out omnidirectionally so that you truly feel the expansive support and tensegrity of your toroidal energy sphere in the universal field. The torus will be discussed more in Chapter 14.

With the help of the Wand*, this chapter's sequence of exercises for specific Perineum Sectors and Press Points of the feet teaches all parts of your perineum to actively engage in the most basic movements of breathing and foot placement that we have already investigated. Keep repeating this series to gain proficiency in the sensing and clamping strength of your entire perineum.

O-RINGS AND DEEP CORE

The perineum is part of the inner tube of O-ring muscles and diaphragms that first develops in the torso of the fetus and houses the yin chi meridians. The O-rings are the basic muscles that a fetus first grows, but when we mature we often forget about them and do not use them voluntarily. They are found in the pelvic floor around the urethra, vagina, uterus and prostate gland in men, at the anus, ileocecal valve and sigmoid colon of the digestive tract, as well as at the heart, veins, arteries, mouth, upper palate, eyes and brain. They are responsible for a lot of automatic functions as well as the release of hormones. However, we can learn to activate some of them voluntarily, as Taoist practitioners have done for thousands of years.

When considering the entire body, these diaphragms are part of the Deep Core connective tissue that actually starts in the arches of your feet between the three Press Points, which Myers (2001) discovered in dissection. For this reason, developing the connection of your feet Press Points with your Perineum Sectors is of prime importance to achieve full internal integration.

The health and functioning of your sexual, reproductive, digestive and urinary systems can be improved by becoming aware of how the musculature of your pelvic floor relates to and integrates with the rest of your body. For a somatic class experience of the pelvic floor and core diaphragms go to the following link: https://mailchi.mp/81a9c144d6f2/perineum-power

Gaining the ability to differentiate and strengthen your perineum will also enable you to reap more profound benefits from the following chapters. In Chapters 11 and 12, you will connect your perineum to two major energy systems:

1. your chakra system, associated with the diaphragms of your inner tube, which pumps energy from your pelvis up to your head and whose first chakra is in the perineum

2. your primovascular chi meridian system and its Twelve Meridian Cycle

DIFFERENTIATE SIX SECTORS

In the figure below, RFPQ stands for Right Front Perineum Quadrant; LFPQ stands for Left Front Perineum Quadrant; RTP stands for Right Transverse Perineal; LTP stands for Left Transverse Perineal; RBPQ stands for Right Back Perineum Quadrant; and LBPQ stands for Left Back Perineum Quadrant.

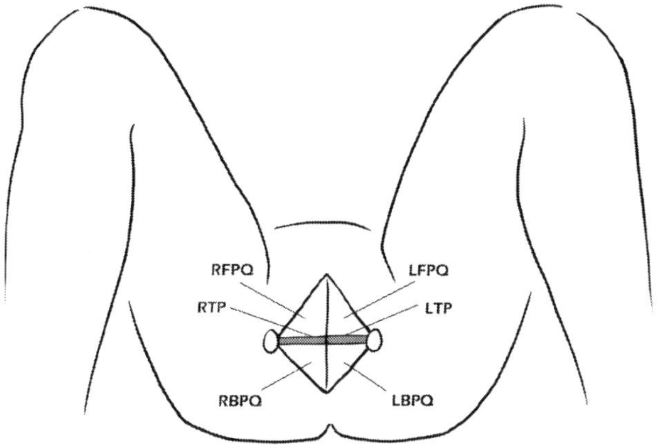

Fig. 13 Perineum Sectors

FRONT PERINEUM QUADRANTS AND PRESS POINTS

We will start at the front perineum and Front Line, as it is the easiest area to access while lying on your back. The front perineum houses both the O-rings of the urethra and the vagina. For illustrations of the Front Lines and front perineum, please refer to Chapter 3.

Left Leg:

- Lie on your back, feet placed hip-width apart as close to your sit bones as is comfortable.
- Lubricate and gently insert the loop of the Perineum Magic Wand into your vagina while inhaling.
- Bend the left loose end so that it comes forward over the left side of your pubic bone to the left of your clitoris, bringing more internal sensation to the left front of your vagina.
- Stage Two Exhale and pull the Wand* inward and upward with your Left Front Perineum Quadrant.
- Repeat until you can feel this Left Front Perineum Quadrant muscle engage effectively on the Wand*.
- Create an Opposing Force by simultaneously pulling outward on the Wand* with one hand and rooting the Big Ball of your left Yang Front

Line a body length into the earth, at the same time as your vagina is drawing upward.

- With this Opposing Force pulling in opposite directions, can you now also sense a Rebound of energy moving up the left side of your inner Yin Front Line toward your spleen and heart?
- Rest (leaving the Wand* inside), breathe freely and feel your energy flow.

Right Leg:

- Repeat with the Right Front Perineum Quadrant and right Big Ball.
- Rest (leaving the Wand* inside), breathe fully and feel your energy. Notice how the slightest conscious touch of your foot Press Point against the earth can instigate a lengthening WAve™ through your inner body.

Both Legs:

- Activate your left and right Front Perineum Quadrants and Big Ball Press Points simultaneously.
- Repeat until you can feel both sides of your vagina engage evenly on the Wand* on the exhale.
- Beach Ball Breathe deeply between repetitions to replenish your energy.
- Rest (leaving the Wand* inside) and sense the increased flow of life force within you.

BACK PERINEUM QUADRANTS AND PRESS POINTS

The back perineum houses the anus O-ring. Be aware that your Yang Back Line forks in three directions at the base of your pelvis: to your left leg and right leg as well as along the tailbone, which is a continuation of your sacrum and spine. For illustrations of the Back Lines, please refer to Chapter 3.

Left Leg:

- If the Perineum Magic Wand is not still inside your vagina, lubricate and gently insert it while inhaling.
- Inhale to fill with chi and, leaving your Big Ball connected to the earth, lift your left Heel up.

- Bend the left loose side of the Wand* so that it goes backward over the Left Back Perineum Quadrant between your tailbone and left sit bone.
- Stage Two Exhale and draw the Wand* upward with your Left Back Perineum Quadrant.
- Repeat until you feel that you can easily clamp on the Wand* while exhaling.
- Create an Opposing Force by exerting a slight pull outward on the Wand* with one hand at the same time as the Heel of your left foot presses the Yang Back Line deeply into the earth.
- Resist this outward pull of hand and foot by drawing upward with your Left Back Perineum Quadrant. Keep your joints soft to feel the Rebound of energy moving up the Yin Back Line along the inside of your spine to your left kidney and creating space between your vertebrae. You may feel the Rebound travel all the way up to the back of your skull as well.
- Rest (leaving the Wand* inside), breathe freely and feel your energy.

Right Leg:

- Repeat with the Right Back Perineum Quadrant.
- Rest (leaving the Wand* inside), breathe fully with all your diaphragms and feel your energy flow.

Both Legs:

- Do the left and right sides simultaneously, grounding through both Heels.
- Place your hands on your buttocks while your Back Perineum Quadrants hug the Wand*.
- Notice if your buttocks and tailbone are also tightening (and in doing so tightening your low back) instead of lengthening. If so, relax them so that you can differentiate their musculature moving downward from that of your perineum moving upward.
- Rest (leaving the Wand* inside), breathe deeply and feel your energy.

Keep practicing this distinction until you can keep your buttocks soft and sit bones and tailbone lengthening downward while simultaneously pulling the Wand* upward with the squeeze of your Back Perineum Quadrants. This perineum practice and general awareness can relieve a lot of tension in your low back and in your bowels.

LATERAL TRANSVERSE PERINEALS AND PRESS POINTS

Although downward movement of the sit bones is a function of the Back Lines, lateral movement of the sit bones is a function of the Lateral Lines and the meaty part of your buttocks is actually on the Yang Lateral Lines. For illustrations of the Lateral Lines, please refer to Chapter 3.

Still lying on your back with your feet placed on the ground close to your hips, reach around and put a hand on each sit bone. As you breathe in and out, can you feel the sit bones expand and come closer together? Notice if their movement apart or together is inhibited.

There is a strong muscle band that goes from the left sit bone to the right sit bone between the vagina and anus, which is called the Transverse Perineal or anatomical perineum. The Transverse Perineal is an amazing muscle! Massaged by a midwife during birthing, it can stretch and expand sufficiently to allow a whole baby to enter the world through this gateway. If it rips during birthing from lack of massage, it will repair on its own! (However, if the surgical cutting of an episiotomy is performed, it does not heal as perfectly.)

Left Lateral Side:

- If the Wand* is not still inside your vagina, lubricate and gently insert it while inhaling.
- Let your inner thighs V outward slightly.
- Bend the left loose end of the Perineum Magic Wand to the left along the inner left thigh, feeling it moving internally toward your left sit bone and contacting the left side of the Transverse Perineal.
- While inhaling to widen and fill with life force, leave the left Big Ball and Heel connected to the earth and lift the left Small Ball off the ground as much as possible.
- Stage Two Exhale and root through the left Small Ball of the left Yang Lateral Line into the earth. Simultaneously exert a slight pull to the left with the left loose end of the Wand*, as if you are about to pull the Wand* out of yourself.
- Create an Opposing Force against the grounding of your Small Ball Press Point and against the outward pull of the Wand* by drawing upward with your Left Transverse Perineal. Keep your joints soft to feel the Rebound move up your left Yin Lateral Line and create space along the fascia that is inside your pelvic girdle, rib cage and jaw.

- Rest (leaving the Wand* inside), breathe freely and feel your energy flowing.

Right Lateral Side:

- Repeat with your Right Transverse Perineal, grounding through the right Small Ball.
- The Opposing Force will send a Rebound of energy up to your liver and right lung.
- Rest (leaving the Wand* inside), breathe and feel your energy.

Both Lateral Sides:

- As you Beach Ball Inhale, feel as if your Yang Lateral Lines are smiling widely. Feel that broadening breath and smile expand your body inside your sit bones, hip bones, rib cage, collarbones and cheekbones.
- As you exhale, contract the left and right Transverse Perineals upward against the pressure of the two sides of the Wand* pulling outward. Simultaneously root through both Small Balls. When the Transverse Perineals are contracted, it feels like their doming is also trying to bring the widened sit bones toward each other, creating Opposing Force and fluid space in the sacroiliac joints.
- Rest (leaving the Wand* inside), breathe freely with all your diaphragms and feel your energy.

FRONT, BACK AND LATERAL SIDES TOGETHER

Stage Three Breathing:

After a Beach Ball inhale to fill with life force, do all these four steps *simultaneously on an exhale*, either physically or with ideokinesis.

1. Imagine light flowing down all your outer body Yang Lines from your head to your feet.
2. Root the Press Points of your Yang Lines a body length into the earth.
3. Clamp on the Wand* with the entire perineum and draw upward toward the other yin diaphragms on the central energy channel, passing the lift of energy to them, like locks on a canal passing a water wave upward.

4. Gently pull outward manually on the Wand* to create more Opposing Force and feel a Rebound increase the lift of the diaphragms of your central energy channel, without any effort on their part.

Activating all four forces *simultaneously* while exhaling will create an omnidirectional and omnidimensional Somatic WAve™ of energy throughout your body. As a result, you may experience yourself expanding beyond your physical body as a continuum of energy connected with the Universal Field.

You will be able to step out of your Perineum Power practice feeling "at one with all that is" and, at the same time, you will have a sense of being grounded and centered in your tan tien and fully functional in earth time. This energetic presence can augment your personal power as well as your impact on the world.

You can also use this energy field for self-healing, as we will now explore in Chapters 11 and 12.

11
AWARENESS OF THE DEEP CORE

Your perineum is part of the inner tube of diaphragms that developed in the fetus. As cells multiplied and created horizontal pumps along the inner tube from the base of your pelvis to the sheath around your brain, the first in-and-out movement pattern of the original cell pulsing at the navel region developed into peristalsis—the involuntary constriction and relaxation of muscles that creates wavelike movements (Keleman, 1985). This Deep Core inner tube houses the chakra system and the yin chi meridians.

Just as you felt the arches activated between the bony Press Point prominences of the base of your feet in Chapter 9, the perineum is the membrane whose dome pulsates among the pubis, sit bones and tailbone, as we just explored in Chapter 10. The illustration to the right was provided with the kind permission of Center Press (Keleman, 1985, p. 45).

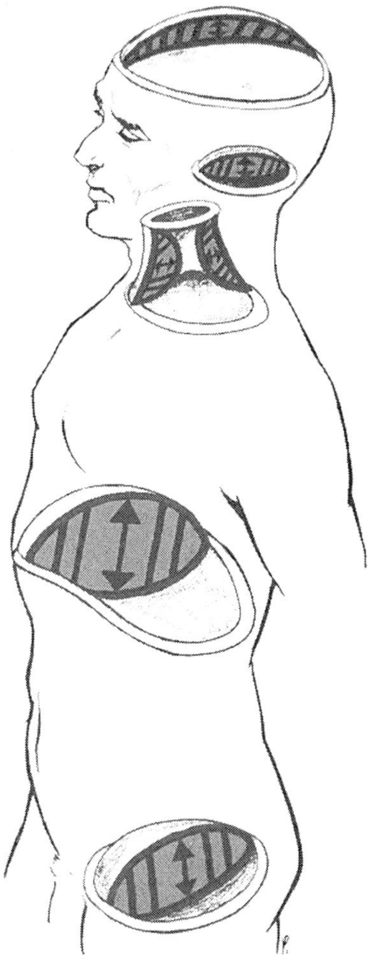

Fig.15 Keleman Diaphragms

DEEP CORE DIAPHRAGMS

CHAKRAS

Each diaphragm of your Deep Core is a thin horizontal sheet of muscle that moves breath and physical substance throughout your body and also enables each of the seven major chakras (energy centers) to take in, incorporate, emanate and pass on energy to the rest of your body.

Chakras are energy vortices of the etheric body that correspond to the location of major hormonal endocrine glands in the physical body. Their activation at progressive stages of evolution can be enhanced by physical movement, mindful breathing practices, transmission of energy and spiritual growth. In traditional yogic practice, bandha energy locks are used for this purpose.

For a healing guided meditation on the chakras and auric field go to the following link: https://mailchi.mp/81a9c144d6f2/perineum-power

DEEP CORE PERISTALSIS

We will now examine a progressive voluntary peristalsis up your Deep Core diaphragms with the following slow, felt-sense exhalation, done with the help of ideokinesis.

- As the perineum domes up, feel this tightening connected to the peritoneum (the membrane that continues from the perineum to envelop your abdominal organs) drawing inward and upward away from the outer walls of your abdominal cavity, creating space between the vertebrae along your spine, like a rolling pin rolling dough upward. The peritoneum connects to the thoracic outlet diaphragm, doming upward like an umbrella opening under your lungs to empty them as you exhale.
- Feel the thoracic diaphragm on top of your lungs contracting downward on the exhale like a heavy cape, pushing air and chi out of your upper lungs up your throat as well as pushing some of the energy out your armpits down your inner arms.
- The rest of the peristaltic wave moves up the tissues of your inner throat through the pharyngeal diaphragm, lengthening your neck so that it feels like a turtle's neck coming out of its shell.

- Feel the doming in the roof of your mouth creating a "yawn without yawning" sensation in the soft tissues at the back of your throat. This "yawn" fountains movement, energy and cerebral spinal fluid up into your brain. You may feel the subtle expansion of your ear canals and plates of your skull, or hear the slight ticks and clicks as the skull plates adjust.

- Another way to access this doming movement into the brain is to place your thumb in your mouth and suck it; you will feel this upward "shwung" rising from your perineum. This whole inner tube is connected from the perineum to the brain—one of the reasons why oral sex can be orgasmic and satisfying for the giver as well.

A more advanced method of O-ring activation of the brain can be practiced when you are ready. You will intensify the "yawn without yawning" effect on the brain by activating the O-rings of the face and eyes as well. This will add even greater well-being to the brain's hypothalamus, where the pituitary and pineal master glands are housed. Taoist practitioners call this part of the brain The Crystal Room and use an Inner Smile to send health-enhancing benefits to the whole body from here, as we did in Chapter 6.

Advanced Activation:

- Drop your lower jaw while forming a tight, long 0 with your mouth and drawing the upper and lower lips firmly into the mouth around the upper and lower teeth; feel how this strongly engages the muscles of the mouth and cheeks. Balance the activation of the left and right sides of your face equally.

- Hold this long 0 formation and simultaneously smile widely with the cheekbones, feeling how this smile starts to lift your upper palate even higher and also adds the emotional benefit of a truly felt smile of appreciation to the hormonal glands. Keep holding.

- To add even greater benefits to the brain's hypothalamus, simultaneously activate the O-ring muscles around the upper and lower eye sockets by closing the eyes, looking downward with the eyeballs and then back toward the center of the head where these glands are located. You can even squeeze the small O-rings of the irises to keep them pliable and to benefit your vision.

- Keep breathing deeply while you hold this formation for as long as you can. You will feel saliva flow increasing and an inexorable desire to yawn, which you should withhold as long as possible in order to keep feeding the hypothalamus with the squeeze of your O-rings, the prana of your breath and your conscious smiling attention.

- When you cannot hold it back any longer, let the yawn flush upward with deep satisfaction.

This progressive standing wave contraction has not only lifted energy up your yin chi meridians and chakra system; it has also massaged spinal fluid from your sacrum up the dural sheath into your brain. You have just created the peristaltic movement up your Deep Core physically, unidirectionally and perhaps quite forcefully with the larger diaphragms. As you learn to initiate it as a Somatic WAve™ of anti-gravity rebounding from the earth and steered by means of Press Points and Perineum Sectors, it will be subtler and more omnidirectional.

SKELETAL ALIGNMENT

These chi meridians run along the riverbeds of our body's system of connective tissue. In his groundbreaking manual, Anatomy Trains, Dr. Thomas W. Myers (2001) reveals a new approach to muscles. Rather than treating muscles as single entities, he views them as being part of twelve myofascial continuities that run in conjunction with the six yang meridians from head to foot as well as with the six yin meridians from foot to head.

Activating the movement of each continuity with muscles is one possibility. Activating the continuity through visualization works in the subtler, albeit just as real, realm of energy. You have recourse to both systems.

Initially, you may want to work purely in the physical realm and, because this trains you in the felt-sense of the Lines of your soma, you will find yourself naturally gaining more profound results as the realm of visualization and energy develops. The more you meditate and visualize energy, the more you will develop the creative healing faculties of your third eye chakra.

You may find that connecting the myofascial continuities of the Yang and Yin Lines to your feet and perineum can release restrictions in movement and bring health to connective tissue and skeletal joints. Using the Perineum Magic Wand to bring awareness and alignment to their flow through the shoulders, back, sacroiliac and hip joints can be very healing.

When I suffered a pelvic and pubic bone separation in a forest accident, this was how I was able to train my inner musculature, with the help of Wand* exercises, to support and align my pelvis and spine from the inside until my ligaments healed. More recently, when I tore four tendons in my left shoulder's rotator cuff, I added regular visualization of the Twelve Meridian Cycle through my shoulder while doing physiotherapy and perineum exercises, which made it possible for me to regain the function of my arm without the two surgeries that had been recommended.

HYDRATION IS IMPORTANT

If you are using your Wand* for alignment purposes, make sure that you have drunk enough water to hydrate your body. Intervertebral discs naturally rehydrate when lying horizontally, if you have enough water in your system.

Your interstitial fluid also needs enough water to allow conduction of energy through the chi meridians of the connective tissue that joins all of your joints in a longitudinal pathway. For more information about this new approach to anatomy, which treats muscles as part of a full body length myofascial continuity rather than individually, please refer to the work of Myers (2001).

STEM CELL FLOW

Besides exercising, aligning, interlacing and balancing your internal musculature and skeletal structure, the six areas of your perineum form the major pump that transports health to your internal organs. The Front Perineum Quadrants activate the spleen meridian connecting to the heart meridian; the Back Perineum Quadrants activate kidney to pericardium meridians; and the Transverse Perineals activate liver to lung channels. However, unless you are working on a specific issue, it is not necessary to know which chi meridian each section of your perineum activates. Just do all the perineum *asanas* (yogic postures) for their overall benefits!

A chi meridian, as well as being an energy pathway, is actually part of a system of fine tubular structures. Korean scientists studying oriental medicine with biophysical methods injected a special staining dye that coloured the meridians. The researchers discovered that the meridian lines are not confined to the skin but are, in fact, a concrete duct system through which liquid flows, and that this liquid aggregates to form stem cells (Yung, 2004).

This is a very exciting discovery that adds another dimension to the potential of who we are and how we can enhance our well-being with stem cells.

On a personal note, my daily use of visualization through the Twelve Meridian Cycle, several times a day for over a year to heal torn shoulder tendons, may also have achieved other benefits. The chi pathways that flow through the shoulder also naturally cycle through the perineum and reproductive organs. My shoulder healing coincided with an "all clear" report from my gynecologist, although checkups in previous years had shown squamous cell irregularities.

RE-EDUCATE AND RE-ALIGN JOINTS

Be patient while initiating the re-education of your muscles. With practice, it is possible to use your Perineum Magic Wand to bring space, traction and healing to the joints of your feet, legs, hip sockets, sacroiliac, lumbar and thoracic spine, shoulders, arms, neck and skull. Recognize how long it has taken you to develop the condition you are addressing now and be willing to release the stress inherent in expecting it to be fixed right away. Stress is one of the psychological factors that creates contraction in this part of your body, whereas joints need to be spacious in order to allow healing stem cell fluid and energy to flow through them.

> "infinite time and no ambition."
>
> *Vanda Scaravelli*

Working with foot Press Point exercises alone will not only strengthen and transform your feet, but also your whole body. The way that your feet meet the ground determines how your posture shifts all the way up to your head as well as how piezoelectricity flows upward to build your bones. Many knee and hip issues can disappear over time when you align your feet properly.

Make sure that you maintain a state of relaxation in the thick short muscles that attach your legs to your hip sockets at the back, sides and front, especially when doing the Perineum Power practices. This will enable your legs to float out toward the Press Points of your feet on the exhale. Similarly, relax the muscles around your knees as you ground through the Press Points to allow space, strengthening and healing into your knee joints. It is important to keep your skeleton "free-floating in a sea of soft tissue," as Dr. Kaparo often reminded us in her Somatic Learning workshops.

Keep your anus and buttocks relaxed when engaging the Back Line so that the tailbone and the energetic extension of your tailbone (which I will call "tail" in order to distinguish it) can lengthen out and entrain your entire low back into traction. Feel the traction going all the way to where your psoas muscles (that lift your legs) internally attach along your spine to your back bottom ribs. Similarly, keep your buttocks relaxed to allow the Lateral Lines to create equipoise in the sacroiliac joints.

Drink water and rest in a horizontal position after your sessions to allow the inner fibers to readjust without the added strain of upright posture. If you have initiated a profound realignment, go to sleep. When you wake up, do the deep breathing of Stages One and Two and repeat your process to deliver more internal space to any stuck places. Once again, rest in a horizontal position after this treatment, allowing time for the connective tissue and intervertebral discs to rehydrate.

Chapters 1 through 11 have already given you the means to:

- bring awareness to the connection between your pelvic floor muscles and breathing
- receive the benefits of improved full breathing practices
- bring awareness and strength to your pelvic floor
- improve sensual and erotic response through this somatic awareness
- bring more health to your inner organs and joints
- create standing waves of support that lift and align your body
- engage your perineum and feet to self-align your pelvis and low back
- enhance your personal power and sacred female vibratory presence on Earth
- make and use a Perineum Magic Wand of Empowerment!

If you also wish to explore more in the realm of self-healing with energy visualization and sensing, continue on to Chapter 12, Ideokinesis.

However, as I mentioned from the onset, it is not necessary to do so immediately, or ever. You have plenty to play with already. Enjoy!

12
IDEOKINESIS

Before continuing to the summation of all the principles that we have been slowly developing, I would like to stoke your imagination with some visualizations that may make your experience more powerful somatically. When using ideokinesis (imaging creates physical movement) to create a Somatic WAve™ Rebound of energy, strength, elongation and alignment throughout your body, it is most effective if you use imagery that is familiar to you. Here are a few possibilities.

CLOTHESLINE

If you have ever hung your laundry out to dry on a traditional clothesline with a pulley at each end, or you are familiar with a flagpole mechanism, this may work for you! This is the image that my students have liked the most.

Either standing or lying down, imagine that a clothesline is moving through the connective tissue of one of your Yang Lines to a clothesline pulley that is located at what I have been referring to as the Push-away Point, at least a body length beyond the Press Point of your Line. As the yang side of the clothesline is pulled on one side, on the other side of the pulley the clothesline is going up the reciprocal Yin Line of your inner body.

With the Wand*:

- As you manually pull outward with the Perineum Magic Wand to create more Opposing Force, imagine that the Wand* is part of the Yang Line moving toward the clothesline pulley positioned at the Push-away Point beyond your Press Point.

- Resist the outward pull with an upward draw of the Perineum Sector that is on the Yin Line counterpart.
- The Yin Line continues up your Deep Core to another pulley beyond your head in the Universal Field, from which it returns as the reciprocal Yang Line flowing through your external connective tissue.

This will help to exercise your pelvic floor. It will also create a strong Rebound that moves up through the inner body diaphragms toward your head and beyond—a continual loop lifting you like laundry floating on the wind, bringing elongation to muscles and joints and chi to the affiliated organs.

WATERPUMP

Just as in the Taoist Yin-Yang symbol, each half contains a dot of its opposite colour, so it is with the breath and water pumping. The full exhale naturally contains the seed of the next inhale within it.

Remember the old water pumps in which you pumped air down a hose into a well that then pushed the water up a pipe to you? Take a full expanding, energizing breath in, and as you exhale down a chosen Line, imagine that you are pushing air down a pipe, which is then forcing a gush of yin energy up into you, supporting your joints from within and washing your corresponding organs with stem cell fluid.

Repeat with the Wand* as explained above for greater perineum strengthening and inner gush.

OCEAN WAVE

This visualization is particularly potent for me, perhaps because I love watching the ocean and floating in the waves.

Imagine that you are easily floating on the surface of a warm sea with your feet pointed toward the shore and your head toward the deep ocean. You are lying at a place on the ocean where the incoming water hits a sandbar on the ocean floor, causing waves to crest. A wave washes over you from the ocean at the same time as you exhale, and your exhale follows the ocean wave moving over your Yang Line toward the seashore. The edge of the wave hits the shore at the same time as the backwash is pulling back toward the ocean depths under the cresting wave where you lie. Feel the backwash moving up through the Yin Line of your inner core diaphragms *at the same time* as the wave is washing over the surface of your body and hitting the shore.

INNER EYE

> "Consciousness is light—
> not a light that can be seen
> with the eyes, but the light
> by which the eyes see."
>
> *Swami Shantananda*

As explained earlier, the perineum is one of the O-ring muscles of the body. The cornea of the eyes as well as the eyelids are also O-rings. Contracting the eyes is one of the techniques recommended by physiotherapists to train the urethral O-ring opening to imitate this easy movement of the eyes in order to treat urinary incontinence. This anatomical fact also makes the following visualization very powerful.

Imagine an eye in the center of your anatomical perineum. As you inhale and the perineum expands outward with the whole inner tube, imagine that this eye is looking outward toward your feet, receiving energy.

As you exhale, feel its eyelids and cornea contract and look inward and upward, bringing the received energy all the way up your Deep Core until it connects with the third eye center for meditation in the hypothalamus of your head, which I have coined the D*-spot (D* being short for *dhyana*, which is Sanskrit for meditation). The combined energies they hold can magnify your presence here.

The "eye" can also continue looking out the top of your head to bring these combined energies out into the perpetual circulating fountain of the toroidal energy sphere that surrounds you and connects you with the Universal Field. I especially like to do this with my feet grounding and physical eyes closed in a meditative state. I call this process Connecting the G-spot with the D*-spot, travelling from the sexual center through the O-rings of the body to the center of consciousness and beyond, experiencing union of body, mind and spirit with All That Is. G-O-D*

Throughout the day, if the perineum is lax, it feels as if the eye is looking down toward your feet. Simply turn it to look inward and upward through the O-rings of your whole Deep Core while maintaining your grounding, and it will create the perfect amount of muscular tone, somatic presence and third eye consciousness to connect your central energy channel both internally and with the Universal Field of which you are a part.

13
INTEGRATION AND UNION

"Allow your life experience to be lightly dusted in form."

Barbara Ann Brennan

The exercises in the next three chapters will summarize and continue to develop the vast holistic healing potential available in the Back, Front and Lateral Lines by consciously connecting chi meridians to the feet and perineum, as well as to the Twelve Meridian Cycle. We will continue to work more in the realm of visualization and ideokinesis as well as felt-sense.

The feet Press Points that we have been grounding and strengthening have connected our yang meridians to the earth and anti-gravity. Staying grounded is one of the best things we can do for our general health and well-being. If climate affords this luxury, doing these exercises with bare feet on the bare earth amplifies the "earthing" benefits even more (Chevalier et al., 2012).

Moving our body helps energy to move. The Perineum Sectors that we have been muscularly moving and developing are now more able to magnify the energetic Rebound of anti-gravity and surf it into health-enhancing yin meridians. Recognize that energy is the underlying force of everything in the Universe. Making energy more coherent inside of us, as well as connected to the earth and cosmic fields outside of us, is a logical recipe for greater health.

TWELVE MERIDIAN INTEGRATION

Although meridians interconnect deep within the torso, they are described as yang or yin depending on their direction of flow either on the surface or on an inner plane of the body. They move in one unbroken chain, with no beginning or end. Their physical basis is the primovascular system; this is a fine tubular network that forms ten hours after fertilization, prior to the cardiovascular and neural systems that it continues to dominate and control throughout our life (Yung, 2004).

The Nobel Prize was awarded to American scientists who proved the molecular basis for circadian rhythms in 2017. However for thousands of years Taoists recognized that there is a biorhythm in nature as well as in our bodies.

Although the yang and yin flows continually cycle through all of our twelve major organ meridians, each meridian naturally takes the lead for two hours in every twenty-four hour period, as shown on the Twelve Meridian Cycle below. This creates an energy rise in the organ, allowing it to do its best work during that two-hour period.

In the following Twelve Meridian Cycle illustration:
AL = Arm Line,
LL = Lateral Line, SB = Small Ball, TP = Transverse Perineal,
FL = Front Line, BB = Big Ball, FPQ = Front Perineum Quadrant,
BL = Back Line, H = Heel, BPQ = Back Perineum Quadrant

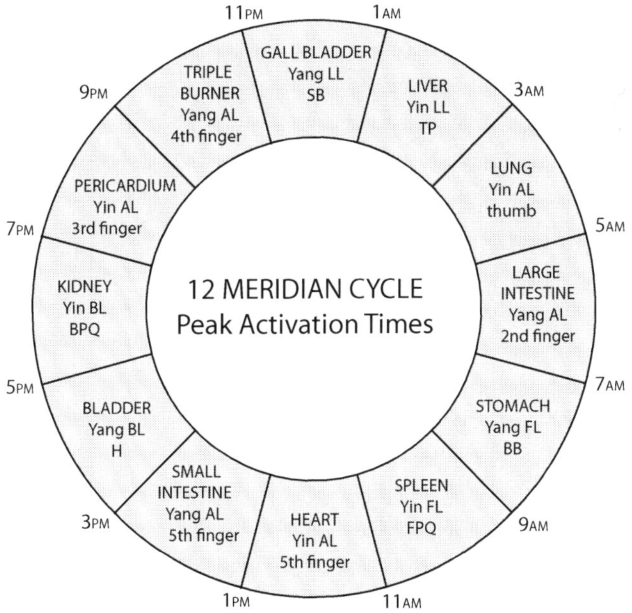

Fig. 16 Twelve Meridian Cycle

When we live in ways that allow our inner organs to be either active or to rest and replenish at the right time, nature supports us and our health benefits.

> Sometimes, though, the life we lead and the abuses we heap upon our bodies cause stress, and sometimes the stress is so intense or so constant that, in effect, it "overloads" the circuit. The "circuit breaker" pops, and needs to be reset before energy can flow properly (Thie, 1994, p.19).

Fortunately the flow of energy can be enhanced:

- by movement
- by stroking with a hand in the direction of flow
- by visualizing energy flowing along the Line with or without movement
- by therapies such as acupressure and acupuncture

Although an organ's function is highlighted at a particular time within a twenty-four hour day, ideally the meridians are continually flowing through the entire circuit, nurturing, integrating and balancing both these organ functions as well as the connective tissues and muscles that the chi meridians flow through. Please become familiar with the continual route of these twelve meridians through your body. Visualize their flow in contemplative meditation with the breath. This circuit will bring vitality, health and healing to your entire physical and emotional body.

The healing of muscles, fascia, joints and organs will be supported. The enhanced flow of chi meridian channels, stem cell fluid and cerebrospinal fluid will bring greater well-being to your entire inner landscape. It is so transformative that your body may tell you to enjoy a nap afterward so that your physical set point can realign with this ideal state of energy flow.

FOLLOW THE TWELVE MERIDIAN PATHWAY

The following three pages are useful to keep highlighted as a summary of the continual pathway of the pairs of yang and yin meridians through the Front, Back and Lateral Lines of the body. Each page starts with the connection of a Yang arm Line to a Yang torso Line, which then Rebounds as a Yin torso Line flowing into a Yin arm Line that will join to the Yang arm line of the following page.

Although we will start with the Front Line, you can start the cycle anywhere.

Starting at the tip of the 2nd finger, inhale light and love; visualize and sense it flowing down the outer finger into Large Intestine meridian all the way to the front of the face; exhale it down Stomach meridian Front Line into the earth, Rebounding as Spleen meridian to Heart meridian and through the armpit down inner 5th finger.

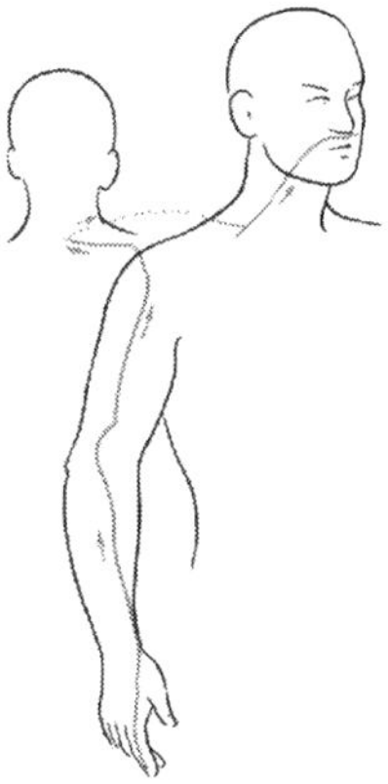

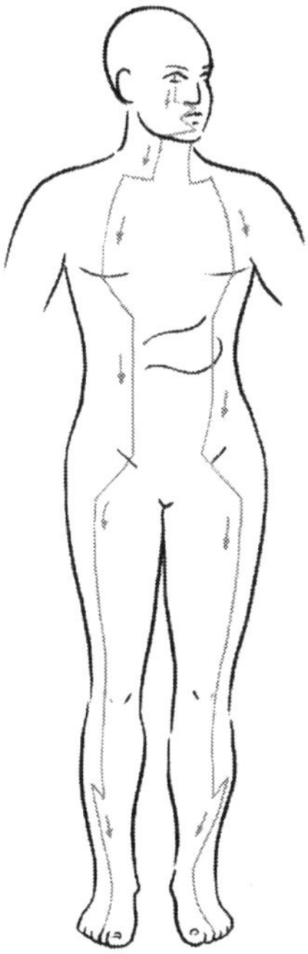

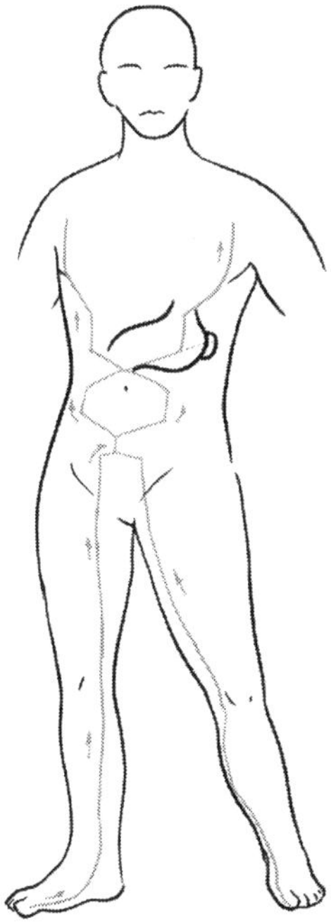

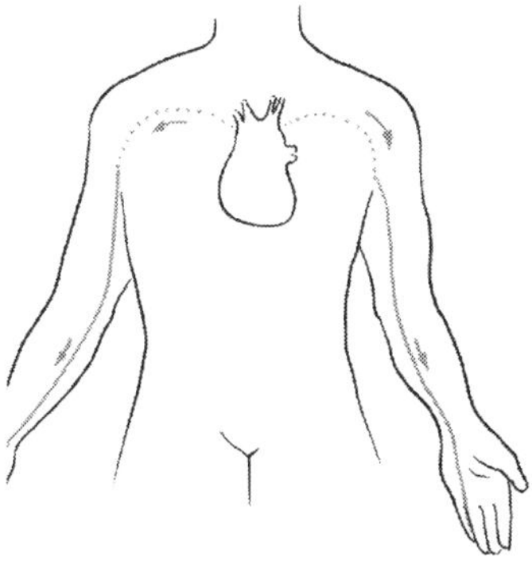

Inhale into the Small Intestine Meridian at the tip of the 5th finger along the outer finger to the side of the face and connecting to Bladder meridian at the front brow; exhale down the Bladder meridian Back Line into the earth, Rebounding as Kidney meridian to Pericardium meridian through the armpit and down inner 3rd finger.

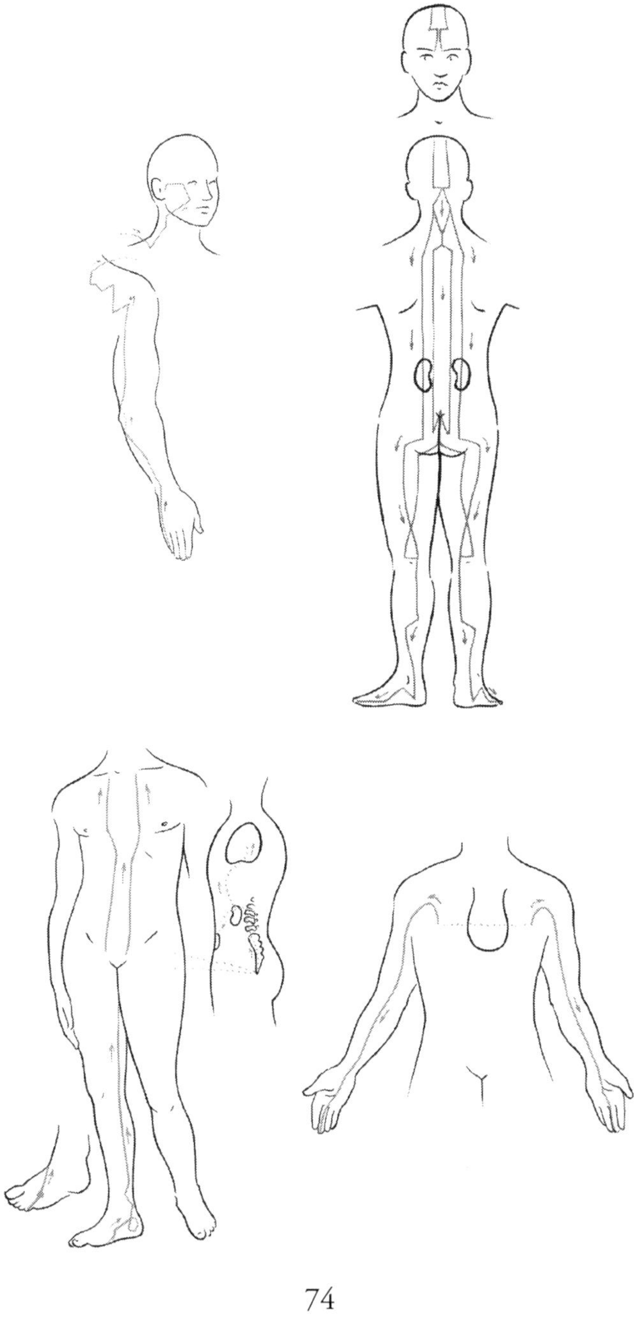

Inhale into the Triple Warmer meridian at the tip of the 4th finger and along the outer finger to the side of the face; exhale down Gall Bladder meridian Lateral Line into the earth, Rebounding as Liver meridian to Lung meridian through the armpit and down inner arm to the tip of the thumb to start again.

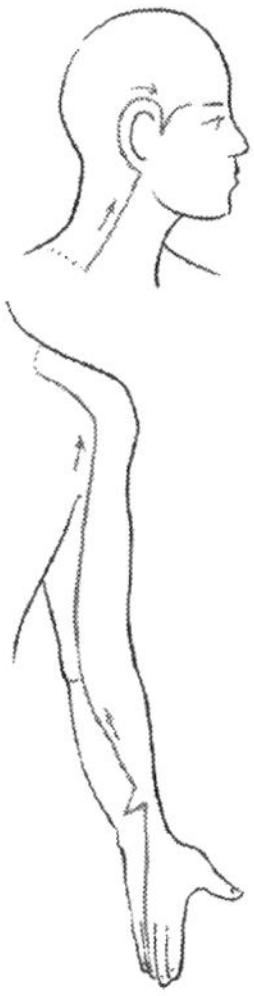

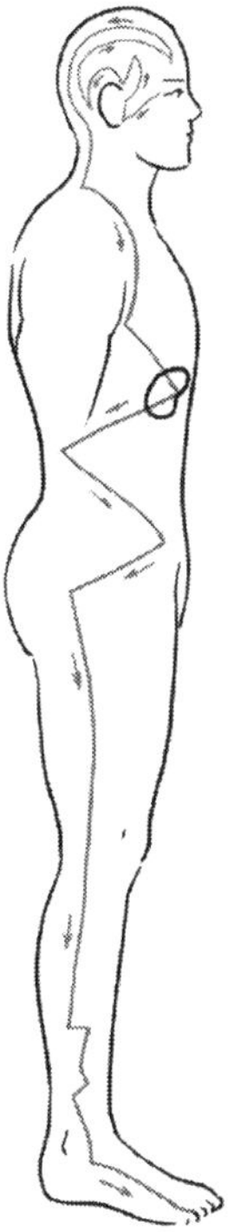

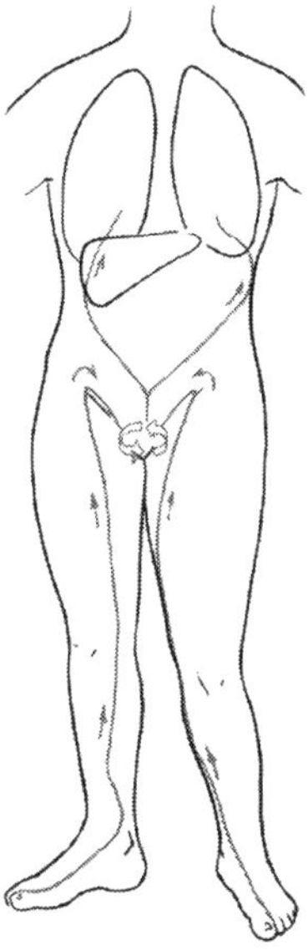

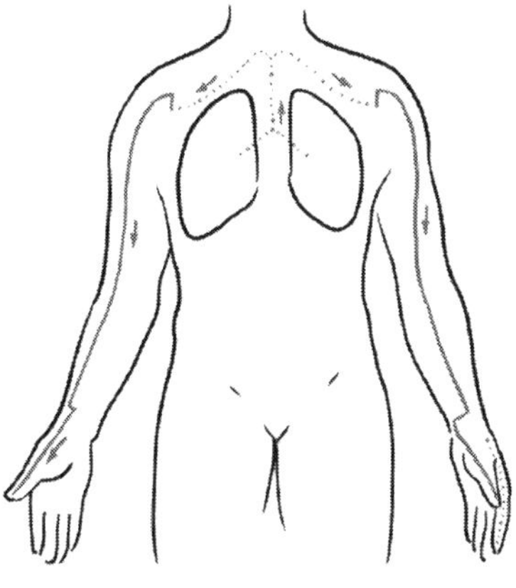

Now that you are familiar with the pathway, enter into a contemplative state with more attention to the breathing of your pelvic floor. By activating your perineum along with the felt-sense visualization of the continual Twelve Meridian Cycle in the following exercise, you will facilitate a depth of personal bodywork for yourself that is quite astounding. The resulting sensation of integration and wholeness in your internal systems is a unique gift that only you can give to yourself.

CONTEMPLATION WITH MUDRA

Join your hands in the classical Indian "Mudra of Innocence" by connecting the two index fingers and thumbs to form a large triangle that you place over your tan tien. Breathe fully and imagine yourself filling with Light. Initially, just spend time breathing in and out and focusing here.

On a physical level, feel the opening of expansive breath in your belly rise into your hands, into the mobility of your sacroiliac joints, into your digestive fire and into the innate vigour of your sexual glands.

On an energy level, all your yin meridians cross here. Follow the pathway of the twelve meridians through this Sea of Energy and throughout your body while your perineum pumps the waves of life force that are your birthright. Visualize and sense. Eventually you will be able to increase the accuracy and speed of the waves, so that you will be able to go around the whole circuit in seconds if you wish.

Your perineum is the secret gateway and activator that ignites the life force and creativity within your tan tien with its movement. This center is where life began for you; it still possesses the seeds of extraordinary possibilities that your life holds for you, if you are aligned with the original force of your soul's urge.

At times of inner questioning or doubt, tune in to the felt-sense of your gut-level intuition with this Mudra of Innocence. As you contemplate choices and possibilities in life, your soma will give you answers. Notice if it responds with feelings of contraction and tension in your belly, heart and lungs, or does it reply with a sense of expansion, ease and perhaps even exhilaration? When you choose to follow your soma's expansive sensations as guidance, you will feel the knots that have been holding you back in life, start to unravel.

PERINEUM ASANAS

Asana is a Sanskrit term used in yoga meaning "seat or manner of sitting." The Oxford English Dictionary defines yoga as a "discipline, a part of which includes breath control, simple meditation and the adoption of specific bodily postures." As "yoga" literally means "union" in Sanskrit, I find "asana" and "yoga" to be perfect terms to describe the intention of our Perineum Power practice.

In the progression of this book, I have been introducing six basic principles and then building on the exploration of these concepts so that you can gradually embody them more fully, as you would in a class series.

In the following three chapters, all the details of each of the three Lines will be brought together. You may find that some parts of these perineum asanas are reinforcing and deepening experiences that you are already familiar with, and yet it may be that you "hear" something for the first time.

Be willing to meet yourself anew each time, listening inside to your soma and becoming your own teacher. The addition of beautiful music to your practice can add further interesting rhythmic layers as you "go with the flow." Stay in the awareness of the moment. You, too, will be different each time.

14
THE FULL BACK LINE ASANA

Although we usually have more awareness in the front of our bodies where our eyes are located and focused on the outer world, it is beneficial to develop a strong Back Line. Energetic presence in the Back Line of the body creates and radiates a sense of groundedness, strength of character and charisma.

The Back Line houses the bladder and kidney meridians, which are associated with personal depth, creativity, sex and desire for life (Gach, 2020). Similarly, the backs of our chakras relate to our sense of self in each facet of our personality, whereas the front of each chakra relates to its connection with the outer world. This distinction is also mirrored in the anatomy of our nervous system. The posterior fibres of the spinal cord have tracts that transmit our sensory information from the body to our brain for assimilation, whereas the front fibers of the spinal cord carry motor impulses from the brain to our muscles.

THE YANG BACK LINE

Imagine that you have eyes on the back of your head and visualize the Yang Back Bladder Lines pictured here flowing on your own body. With your hands, palpate down your Right and Left Yang Back Lines to increase your somatic awareness. Bring particular awareness to the areas that are usually curved, bent or creased.

Create a sensory connection with the back of your body. Connect to any points on the Lines where you feel an itch, a twinge, a pain, or are simply drawn to them. You are very likely feeling an acupressure point calling to you for stimulation; this was my realization after studying acupressure. Many points have a slight divot in the bone or the musculature. When you hold an acupressure point and deeply breathe into it, your body releases endorphins. Hold it for about three minutes, lightly at first with your fingertip, and gradually deepening the pressure only if it is comfortable. Release the point gradually as well (Gach, 2020). It is beyond the scope of this book to give detailed information about the location of specific acupressure points on the Lines; however, many charts and courses are available on the internet.

Ground Reference Scan:

Start exploring your Yang Back Line and your relationship to gravity with the following Ground Reference Scan based on Somatic Learning (Kaparo, 2003). You will also be repeating this Ground Reference Scan for comparison after doing Perineum Asanas.

- Lie down full length on the floor, facing up.
- Imagine that the back of your body has been painted with a paint roller. What print would you leave on the floor at points of contact? Compare your left and right sides.
- Imagine yourself lying on a soft sandy surface. What imprint would you leave? Compare your left and right sides.

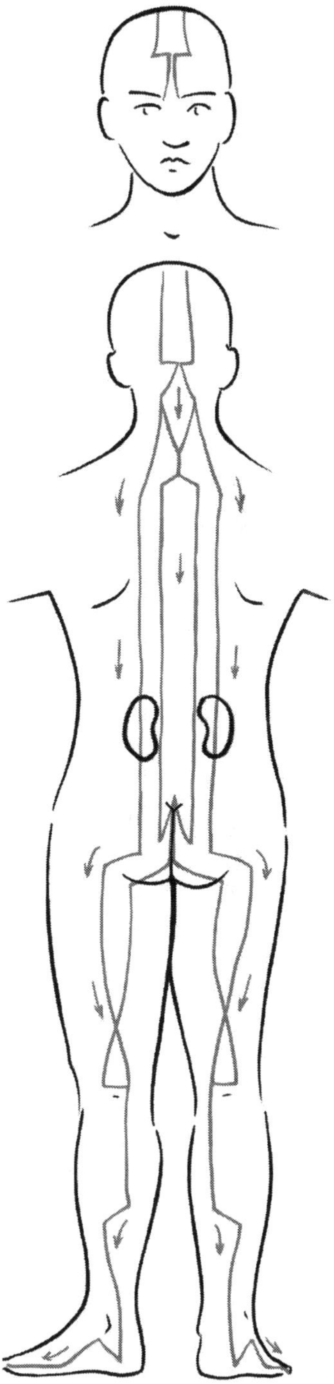

Fig. 2 Yang Bladder Back Line

- Notice the spaces between the backs of your knees and the floor, your low back and the floor, and the tops of your shoulders and the floor. Compare your left and right sides. What creature could crawl through these spaces?

Like the Press Points of the feet, when the back or any part of your body can fully release into gravity through its point of contact, it is naturally lifted upward by anti-gravity and does not have to hold itself up with external skeletal muscles.

YANG AND YIN BACK LINES, PRESS POINTS AND PERINEUM QUADRANTS

Yang Back Line of the Tail:

Be aware that the Back Line forks in three directions at the base of the pelvis: left and right legs continuing from your hip bones, tailbone continuing from your spine.

For an introductory somatic class experience of the Back Line go to the following link in order to deepen this experience with the use of the Wand*: https://mailchi.mp/81a9c144d6f2/perineum-power

- Lie on your back with your knees bent and feet placed hip-width apart close to your buttocks.
- Gently insert the lubricated Perineum Magic Wand while inhaling.
- Bend the loose ends of the Wand* so that they go backward, feeling them toward your anus and tailbone.
- Beach Ball Inhale to fill your entire body with life force.
- Stage Two Exhale: Visualize gold channels of liquid light moving from your skull on each side of your spine to your tailbone.
- Imagine that the exhale that compresses your tan tien releases a force that shoots your tail out like a light balsa raft on this channel of liquid light and turns on an electric winch, at least a body length away, that draws the energetic extending tail toward it.
- Manually exert a slight pull outward on the inserted Wand* in the same direction.

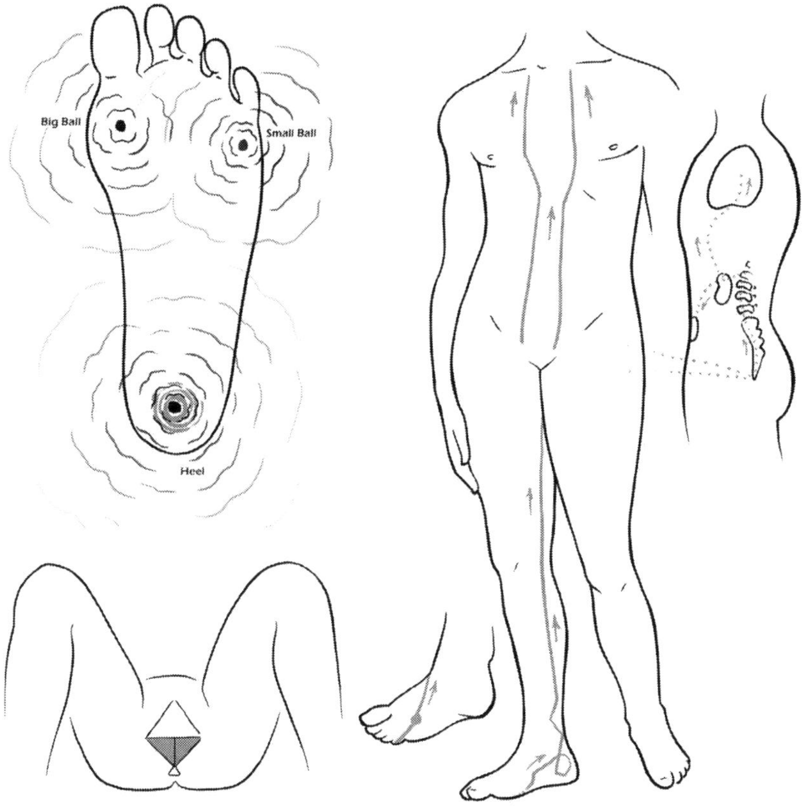

Fig. 17 Components of Back Line Rebound

Yin Back Line of the Tail:

- Simultaneously draw both your Left and Right Back Perineum Quadrants up into your body against the resistance of the winch and Wand* pulling outward, creating an Opposing Force that you will be able to surf.
- Keep buttocks soft.
- Feel a lengthening Somatic WAve™ Rebound all the way up through the connective tissue of the peritoneum into the Yin Kidney Back Line, moving into the kidneys and creating space between the vertebrae of the lumbar and thoracic spine and neck, all the way to your skull.
- Rest (leaving the Wand* inside), breathe and feel your energy.
- Repeat the Ground Reference Scan.

Yang and Yin Back Lines of the Left Leg:

- Inhale to fill with chi and, leaving the ball of the foot connected to the earth, lift the left heel up.
- Stage Two Exhale and imagine a golden channel of liquid light moving from over your skull to the left of your spine, out the left sit bone, down the back of your left leg, and down into the earth as you activate the Heel Press Point and visualize the very center of the heel sending the Yang Line deep into the ground a body length away.
- Use the same visualization as you did for the tailbone above. As you press the Heel into the ground, imagine that a Line is going out your Heel to a winch a body length away from your foot and, when your exhale turns on the winch, it starts pulling the whole Left Yang Back Line toward it.
- Compound the force by physically pulling on the left loose end of the Wand* so that it goes back toward the left side of your anus and tailbone.
- Beach Ball Inhale and Stage Three Exhale: While still exhaling and keeping the buttocks soft and the tail lengthening, resist the outward force by pulling inward and upward with the entire breadth of the Left Back Perineum Quadrant between your tailbone and sit bone.
- This causes a Somatic WAve™ to Rebound along the Left Yin Back Line of the arch of the foot, back of the inner ankle, calf, knee and thigh into the Left Back Perineum Quadrant.
- Pull up with this muscle and feel the elongation of a WAve™ all along the left back side of the Deep Core of connective tissue that connects your perineum to the peritoneum, to the left back side of the thoracic outlet diaphragm, to the kidney, through the left back side of the pleural sheath of the lungs, throat, mouth, upper palate and dural sheath of the brain, while yang energy enters the ground through the Heel.
- Rest (leaving the Wand* inside), breathe and feel your energy.
- Repeat the Ground Reference Scan. Notice the difference in how the back of your body now contacts the floor.

You have experienced the kidney meridian, which is the yin partner to the yang bladder meridian. The kidney meridian then connects to the pericardium meridian that flows out the palm side of your third finger.

Yang and Yin Back Lines of the Right Leg:

- Repeat with the right side of the Yang Back Line grounding through the Heel Press Point, while pulling up the entire breadth of the Right Back Perineum Quadrant and elongating into the Right Yin Back Line.

- Rest (leaving the Wand* inside), breathe and feel your energy.

- Repeat the Ground Reference Scan.

The Full Back Line Asana:

- Stage Three Exhale: Engage all aspects of the Yang and Yin Back Lines together—grounding through the tail along with the left and right Heels, while drawing up with the Back Perineum Quadrants, to surf energy through the entire inner Yin Back Line with a Somatic WAve™.

- Make sure that the buttock muscles remain soft as the yang energy flows through them toward your feet.

- You may notice that your pelvis rises on the lengthening exhale, as if you were starting to do the Bridge Pose in yoga. If so, inhale to refill with energy at the height of the pose, then use another Stage Three Exhale to lower one vertebra at a time, each link coming to the mat and lengthening the connective tissue to the next vertebra with the WAve™ before that vertebra comes down to the mat.

- Rest, breathing freely. Feel your energy.

- Remove the Wand*.

- Repeat the Ground Reference Scan, noting prints, imprints, spaces and the greater contact that you are now making with the floor.

Notice that the more you connect with the ground, the more you can release into gravity, and the more you are lifted up effortlessly by anti-gravity!

- Draw your knees up into your chest, hugging them in and rocking side to side on your low back. Roll over onto one side into a fetal position, continuing to hug yourself and sense internally.

- Slowly push up onto your hands and knees, and then move into a squat (or crouch with your hands holding a chair for balance and support.) Create a connection of your Heels and tail deep into the earth as you prepare to stand. If your heels do not actually touch the floor because of tight calf muscles, initially you may wish to put a block under them in order to have something to press against as you ground your energy into the earth through your feet.

- Beach Ball Inhale and gather energy.
- Stage Three Exhale: Straighten your legs, pressing both Heels deep into the earth, and imagine that you have a gold bowling ball attached to your tail, dropping it into the earth. Simultaneously pull up your Back Perineum Quadrants to create Opposing Force.
- Feel the Rebound shooting all the way up your inner body, effortlessly floating you to a standing position.
- Release this geyser of energy out the top of your head and visualize it showering down the outsides of your body back into the earth, where you once more gather it up through your feet in the perpetual motion of a toroidal energy sphere.

TOROIDAL ENERGY SPHERE

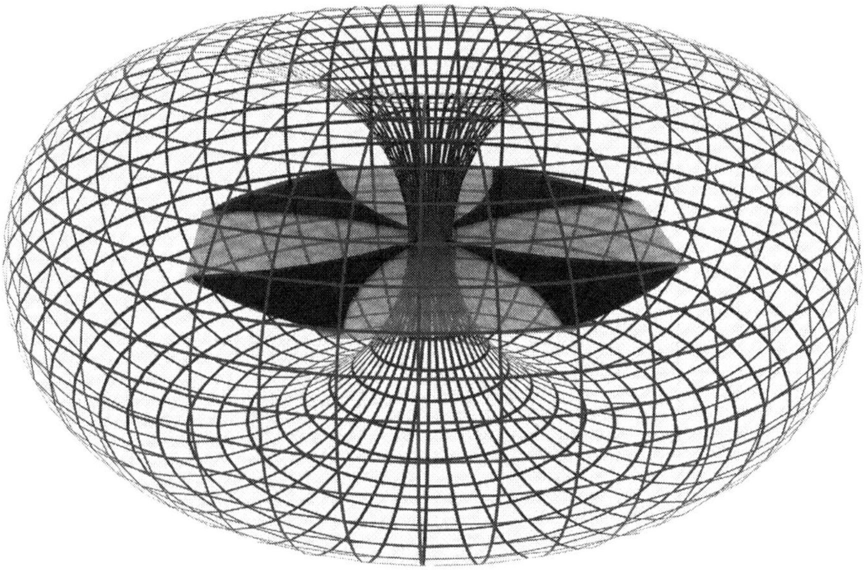

Fig. 18 Toroidal Energy Sphere

The torus is the primary energy pattern that exists in every scale of nature, from a small atom, to the magnetic field around Earth, to the structure of a whirlpool galaxy. Some scientists have suggested that the energy field of Earth, if they could learn how to tap into it, could become a source of free energy for everyone on the planet. It would also be a *clean* source of energy as it does not involve smashing things together (nuclear power) or combustion (oil).

The torus is also the energy field of our bodies, into which we *can* learn to tap.

15
THE FULL FRONT LINE ASANA

The front of the body is our connection to the outer world. An open Front Line communicates "yes" to the world, and a contracted Front Line says "no." Our mouth and eyes orient forward and so we are usually more conscious of our front than we are of our back and lateral sides. For the same reason, we may also find it easier to feel the connection of the Front Lines to their Press Points and Perineum Quadrants than we do in the other Lines. Notice that when babies start to walk upright, they walk on the balls of their feet, and it takes a while for their heels to come down.

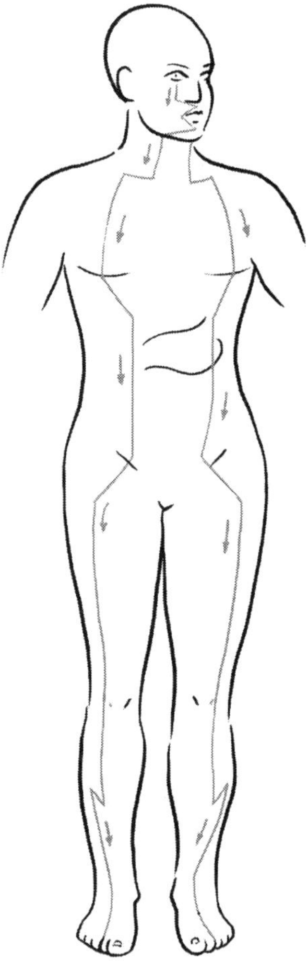

Fig. 4 Yang Stomach Front Line

THE YANG FRONT LINE

With your hands, stroke and palpate down the Left and Right Front Yang Lines that are pictured in the diagram. Create a sensory connection to your Front Lines. Connect to any tender or itchy points by holding and breathing into them. Notice that the pubic bone is on the downward flow of yang energy. People often draw the pubis up with the inner core and cause constriction in their groins.

Yang Front Line of the Left Leg:

- Lie on your back with your knees bent and feet placed hip-width apart close to your buttocks.
- Inhale and gently insert your lubricated Wand*.
- Bend the left loose end so that it comes forward over the left side of your pubic bone, to the left of your clitoris, bringing more internal sensation to the left front of your vagina.
- Stage Three Exhale and exert a slight pull on the left loose end in that position. Resist it by drawing inward and upward with the Left Front Perineum Quadrant.

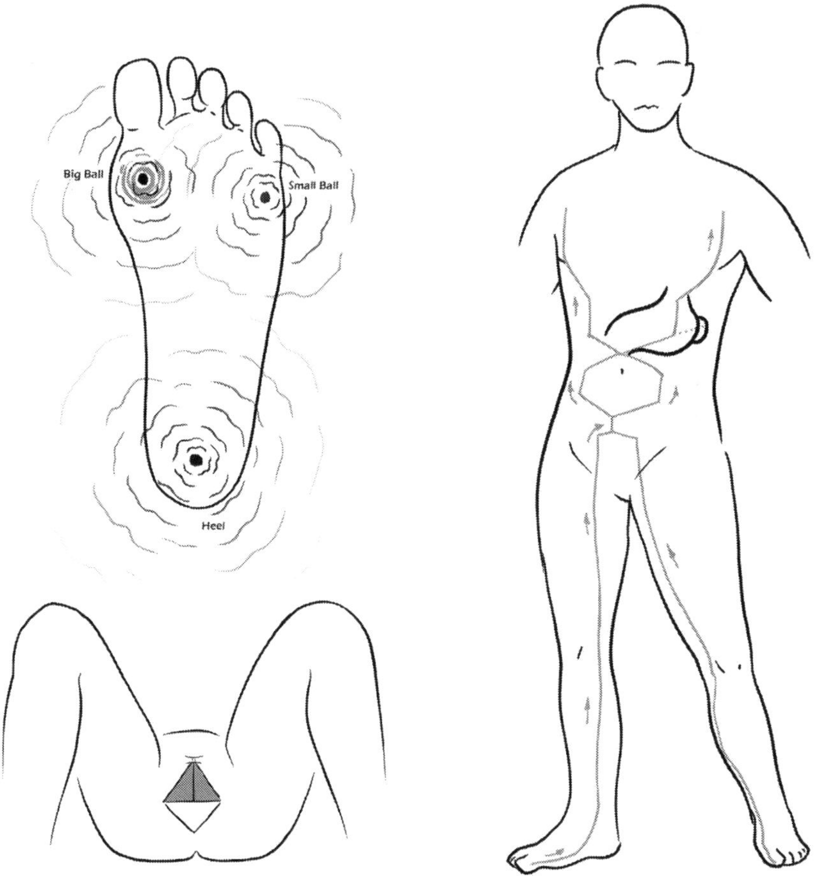

Fig. 19 Components of Front Line Rebound

- Rest (leaving the Wand* inside), breathe freely and feel your energy.
- In order to activate the energy flow, visualize the yang stomach meridian in Fig. 4 on your own body: Imagine and sense a channel of gold liquid light flowing down the surface of your left front body from head to toes, starting at the left cheekbone, continuing down the left side of the throat, through the left nipple, stomach and abdominal muscles to the pubic bone, crossing the inguinal ligament to the front of the left thigh and continuing to the kneecap, shin, front of the ankle, off the toe-foot of the first three toes and rooting through the Left Big Ball Press Point.

THE YIN FRONT LINE

- Imagine the Front Yang Line going a body length into the ground and Rebounding back from the earth as a silver channel of energy that ascends the Yin Front Line along the arch of the inner foot, ankle, knee and thigh into the Left Front Perineum Quadrant, as pictured above in Figure 19.
- Add a physical sensation of gratitude and love to this experience—of being grateful for and loving this earth energy and this body—feeding your heart, coming more mindfully into the here and now.
- Continue to steer the Rebounding yin energy with your Left Front Perineum Quadrant up into the peritoneum, to the spleen, thoracic outlet diaphragm, pleural sheath of the left lung, throat, mouth, upper palate and dural sheath of the brain.
- Rest (leaving the Wand* inside), breathe and feel your energy flow.
- This is, in fact, the yin spleen meridian that then continues to connect to the heart meridian, which flows to the palm side of the baby finger. The spleen is the yin partner to the yang stomach meridian. Together they form the Front Line.

Yang Front Line of the Right Leg:

- Repeat with the right side of the Yang Front Line, pulling up the Right Front Perineum Quadrant into the Yin Front Line while grounding through the Right Big Ball Press Point.
- Rest (leaving the Wand* inside) and replenish with Beach Ball Breath.

The Full Front Line Asana:

- Stage Three Exhale: The gold yang channels flow down the outside of your front body from the cosmos out the Big Balls at the same time as the silver yin channels come Rebounding from the earth up the inner legs and torso.

- Keep the pubic bone descending down the Yang Line so that, when the Front Perineum Quadrants draw up, space is created at the front groins and the front hip sockets are able to decompress. This is one of the wonderful advantages of the Somatic WAve™ method!

- You may notice that in your horizontal position, the front of your pelvis rises somewhat, bowing upward to accommodate this increased space in the front groins. You may also feel your front thigh muscles lengthening effortlessly out your knee joints and creating space therein.

- The deeper you physically press the Big Ball Press Points into the earth (or eventually just visualize them pressing) at the same time as the front triangle of the perineum draws up, the greater is the Opposing Force and the greater is the Somatic WAve™ that Rebounds up your inner body, creating space between joints and lengthening muscles as it goes.

- When you have completed this process, remove the Wand* and rest. Breathe deeply and feel your energy.

- Draw your knees into your chest, hugging them in and rocking side to side on your low back. Roll over onto one side into a fetal position, continuing to hug yourself and sense internally.

- Slowly push up onto your hands and knees, and then move into a squat (or crouch with your hands holding a chair for balance and support) while you feel the connection of your Big Ball Press Points into the earth.

- Beach Ball Inhale and gather energy.

Mirror Ideokinesis:

- Imagine that the floor you are standing on is a mirror.

- Picture the mirror image of yourself beneath the surface of the floor.

- As you stand up and straighten your legs, exhale and visualize energy flowing from your head down the front of your body through the Big Balls *into the mirror image reflected below the floor.*

- See it moving down the front of your feet, ankles, shins, knees, thighs, pelvis, chest, neck and face, to the top of your head below the surface of the mirror.

THE SOMATIC WAVE™

- Keep your attention moving down the imagined image below the surface of the floor, rather than in your physical body above the floor.
- As you do so, you will find yourself zooming upward in your actual physical body while your feet are on the ground, floating effortlessly to an elongated standing position.
- When you first feel the excitement of being lifted, it can be tempting to shift your attention to your physical body; however, if you do so, you will fall off the WAve™.

This splitting of attention can be challenging at first, but it is worth the practice to stay grounded, even when you feel the WAve™ physically lifting you more and more on the Rebound. Strengthening your general ability to stay grounded is very useful, as it can be applied to intense emotional situations as well.

Where attention goes, energy flows.

- Release the energy out the top of your head.
- Feel it showering down the outside of your body back into the earth in the perpetual motion of the yin-yang symbol, like a fountain that then ascends again, turning into an inhale, which turns into an exhale, which turns into an inhale . . . seamlessly self-supporting you in your toroidal energy sphere while you feel yourself physically expanding.

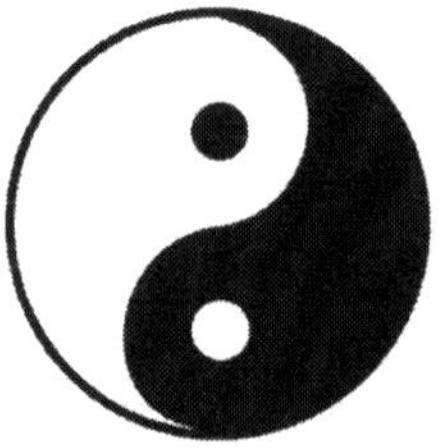

Fig. 21 Yin Yang Symbol

16
THE FULL LATERAL LINE ASANA

Touch and stroke the sides of your body to increase your somatic awareness as you study the diagram on the following page. Look at your side body in a mirror and notice that it is almost as wide as your back or front. We are often unconscious of the full breadth of the sides of our body and do not allow its full expression, as if we were only a two-dimensional paper cutout.

Reach down and palpate your sit bones, noticing how close they are to your tailbone and how narrow they are in terms of the whole configuration of your pelvic bowl. Although downward movement of the sit bones is a function of the Back Lines, lateral movement of the sit bones is a function of the Lateral Lines. The meaty part of your buttocks is actually on a Lateral Line and not on a Back Line, as most people assume.

Notice that the gall bladder meridian goes deep into the side of the buttock, into the area where the very thick sciatic nerve can become impinged by the piriformis muscle. However, if you feel the lateral sides of the sit bones and the Lateral Lines stretching sideward with the activation of the Transverse Perineals, you will expand in this area.

IMPORTANCE OF HIP SWAY

We easily move our hips frontward and backward, rolling our feet from heel to toe as we look forward to where we are going. But we often forget to sway our hips side-to-side with our Lateral Lines, sweeping through the Now more fully, or to engage the Lateral Lines in alternating rotational corkscrew movements of the pelvic and shoulder girdles when we walk.

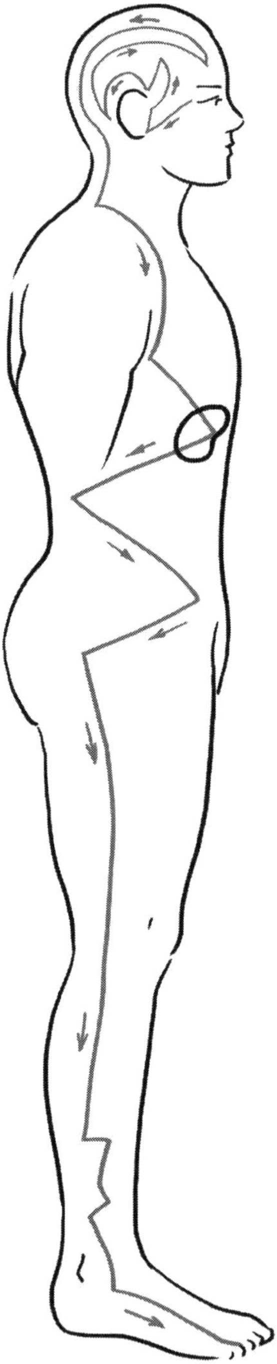

Fig.6 Yang Gall Bladder Lateral Line

Women who have been raised in restrictive cultures seldom allow their pelvis to move in a full fish spine sway when they walk because of this movement's connotations in their society. When Western missionaries and visitors first arrived on the Hawaiian islands, they found the natural health-enhancing movements of the sacred hula to be immoral. Mark Twain described how "at night they feasted and the girls danced the lascivious hula-hula — a dance that is said to exhibit the very perfection of educated motion of limb and arm, hand, head and body" (Mutual Publishing, 2003, p. 15).

Allowing the hips to hang and sway like heavy fruit on a tree is a basic movement that is healthy, not only for the skeleton but also for the brain! Hip sway is an upright continuation of Creeping and Crawling, which is practiced in Nia 5 Stages: Embryonic, Creeping, Crawling, Standing and Walking. It has been found that, if babies do not crawl but go straight to standing, their development of left-right brain integration is hampered; however, they can be retrained in adulthood. "Practiced with awareness, these stages have the power to facilitate optimal alignment, improved function and comfort in the body. This system provides a tool for reclaiming and sustaining mobility, flexibility, strength, agility and stability" (Nia, 2020).

Hip sway is not only healthy for the body and brain; it is also symbolic of relaxed femininity. If the Front Lines say "yes" to the world and turning the back says "no," then the Lateral Lines say "maybe" and "therefore the Lateral Line is often presented in advertisements that want to portray the attitude of seduction" (Myers, 2009, p. 128). You may notice that advertising often depicts a female model looking at you from the side of her body. The subliminal messages that the marketing world has discovered can increase your voluptuary Perineum Power. If you want to relax in your sensuality and keep your hips healthy and moving freely, practice letting them sway side-to-side and experience more space and freedom in your life.

Perhaps any remnants of the centuries of shaming that I spoke of in Chapter 1 are starting to be lifted from you by a new appreciation of the inherent potential in this perineal gateway to creativity, health, sexual bliss, spirituality and cosmic union.

LATERAL LINES, PRESS POINTS AND TRANSVERSE PERINEALS

Left Yang Lateral Line:

- Lie on your back with your knees bent and your feet placed hip-width apart close to your buttocks.
- Gently insert the lubricated Perineum Magic Wand while inhaling.
- Beach Ball Inhale to fill with chi. Leaving the Big Ball and Heel Press Points connected to the floor, lift the Small Ball Press Point up on the inhale.
- Stage Three Exhale and imagine a channel of gold liquid light flowing down the lateral surface of the left side of your body from the side of your head to the blade of your left foot, starting on the left side of your skull just outside the left eye socket, continuing down the left side of the neck, ribs, waist, buttock muscle, outer hip, ilio-tibial band of thigh, knee, calf, outer ankle and blade of the foot, off the baby and fourth toes and grounding into the earth through the Small Ball Press Point as you lower it. This is the left side of the gall bladder meridian.

Left Yin Lateral Line:

- Let your inner thighs V outward slightly. As much as is possible with your hands, sweep them up toward the sit bones of the Yin Lateral Lines shown in the following diagram.

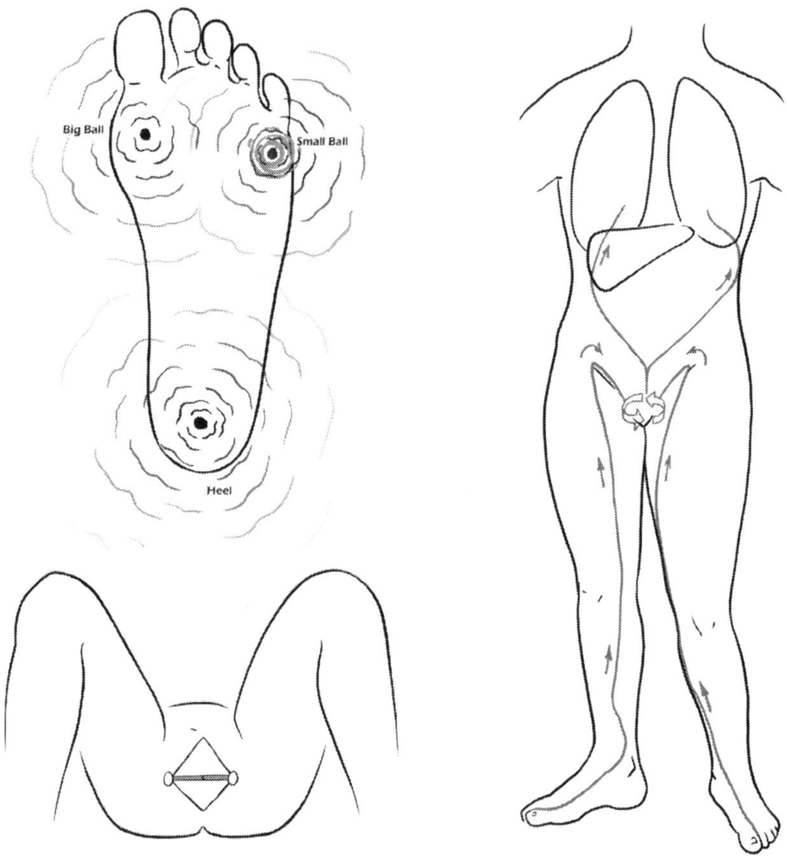

Fig. 20 Components of Lateral Line Rebound

- Bend the left loose end of the Wand* to the left along the inner left thigh, feeling it move internally toward your left sit bone and contacting the left side of the Transverse Perineal.

- Stage Three Exhale and, while grounding the Small Ball of the Yang Lateral Line deep into the earth, exert a slight pull to the left with the loose end of the Wand* and resist it by pulling upward with the Left Transverse Perineal. This creates a Rebound that lengthens up the inside of the inner left lateral pelvis, waist, chest, throat, mouth and jaw to the left ear canal.

This Yin Liver Lateral Line is the yin partner of the Yang Gall Bladder Lateral Line. It then connects to the lung meridian that flows through the armpit and along the inner arm to the palm side of the thumb.

Right Yin Lateral Line:

- Repeat with the right side of the Transverse Perineal, rooting through the Right Small Ball.
- Rest, breathe and feel your energy.

The Full Lateral Line Asana:
Still lying on your back with knees bent, alternately place your left and right foot on the floor and, as you shift your weight from foot to foot, allow your hips to swing side-to-side along the contour of a crescent moon. Notice the slight corkscrew motion of the pelvic girdle as the alternate Transverse Perineals contract toward each sit bone, similar to the agitation action of a washing machine.

- Stabilize both feet on the ground, a full generous hip-width apart, and Stage Three Exhale: Engage all aspects of the Yang and Yin Lateral Lines together—grounding energy down both Yang Lateral Lines through the Left and Right Small Ball Press Points while drawing up the Transverse Perineals to surf energy up both Yin Lateral Lines with the Rebound of a Somatic WAve™.
- Using the previous ideokinetic images of the Eye, Winch, Clothesline, Fountain, Mirror, etc. may facilitate your Rebound.
- Make sure that the outer hip sockets and knee joints remain soft as the yang energy flows through them toward your feet and deep into the earth, so that you will be able to feel the Rebound.
- Rest, breathe and feel your energy.
- Repeat the Ground Reference Scan.

Do a quick body check and notice whether you have added this new awareness of lateral space in order to increase the volume now available to you between the Front and Back Lines as they Rebound back up through their respective Perineum Sectors. You may feel a remarkable spaciousness within your physical vessel.

Inhale and smile widely across your cheek bones. Mimic that wide facial smile and mirror it between your sit bones all the way up your Deep Core to your widening collarbones. When the entire anatomical perineum and Lateral Lines are expanded laterally, it feels like a wide smile is stretching from sit bone to sit bone. Sense whether this feels good to your pelvis and sacroiliac joints. This widening can also be experienced when you are in a seated or standing position, without the Wand*.

SACROILIAC SELF-CARE

Jammed Joint:

If you ever notice that the mobility of one of your sacroiliac joints is jammed, you may be able to use your Lateral Lines to widen your pelvis and unlock it. First, follow the process below with your face so that you can then mimic it with your sacrum:

- Put an exaggerated smile on your face, widening your cheekbones to smile like a Cheshire cat.
- Hold the wide smile but resist it by contracting your mouth, or sucking a thumb up toward your palate, while keeping your cheek bones widened. Can you feel the subtle effect that this has on the back of your neck where it joins your skull?

Your mouth is part of the same inner tube of fascia that starts in your foot arches and continues all the way through the core of your torso and throat to surround your brain. With your Wand* inserted, replicate the cheekbone and mouth experience in the soft tissue between your sit bones:

- Lie on your back with feet placed on the ground close to your hips.
- Place your feet so that your heels turn out more than your toes, which widens your sacrum.
- Inhale to expand your perineum and widen your hip bones apart into a "smile."
- Exhale and send yang energy down the outer hips and legs through the Small Balls into the earth.
- During the same exhale, oppose an outward pull of the Wand* by hugging inward and upward with your yoni and internal pelvic muscles, mirroring how you sucked with your mouth.

This sequence enables your sacrum to move up and away from where it has sunken down between your ilia (back of your hip bones) as they widen. The relationship of your sacrum to your pelvic bowl is like the keystone of a masonry arch that locks all the stones of the arch into position. By drawing the Deep Core perineum and abdominal peritoneum on the visceral surface of your sacrum upward, you may be able to release the stuck wedge.

Keeping your joints soft will enable the Rebound from the Opposing Force to provide even more space and relief. If the condition has been long-standing, be patient in your attempt to gradually strengthen and re-educate your inner muscles to draw upward evenly, while your outer muscles and joints remain soft.

ALL BACK, FRONT AND LATERAL LINES TOGETHER

Three Point Stability:

I mentioned earlier, when explaining the three Press Points of the feet, that a triangle is the most stable geometric shape. This premise can also be applied to becoming aware of the triangle formed by your two feet and tailbone when you are in full perineum asana, either seated or standing, particularly if in sumo stance. In either position, place the feet wide apart under your bent knees so that energy can still travel down your perpendicular shin bones like fence posts into the earth, and sense the energetic extension of the grounding area as your tail forms the back point of the triangle.

Shoulder, Neck and Head Alignment:

As you Beach Ball Inhale, feel your perineum balloon downward and your upper chest expand upward. When you exhale, the bottom and top of your torso move toward your tan tien, the perineum doming upward and the thoracic diaphragm over your lungs pressing downward. Feel how the widening stretch that occurs in the perineum between your sit bones and tailbone, as well as in the low back, is mirrored by the widening stretch of the top of your shoulder muscles between the rotator cuffs (where the arms join the shoulders) and your neck. Both widen with the exhalation.

> "As above, so below."
>
> *Hermes Trismegistus*

Placing your hands with the palms facing down will help you to focus most of your attention on the downward descent of your energetic tail into the mirror image of your tail, back, neck and head beneath the floor so that your physical neck and head will lengthen upward on the Rebound. This will enhance the vertical axis of your spine by helping to send your neck upward in relation to your shoulder girdle, instead of hunching forward off its vertical axis. The extension of your neck and head can also be enhanced by putting the tip of your tongue on the roof of your mouth.

The Cape:

When we grew in utero from the first cell, we initially multiplied into a tubular sheath that then bent from each side of the spinal line to seal in the front at what is called the linea alba (where extremely large bellies of pregnant women can sometimes split apart slightly) to make our front surface. In other words, our side bodies grew from the back toward the front, like a cape wrapping us and then closing.

- Inhale the cosmic light and, with a Stage Three Exhale, recreate this image of a cape wrapping your body in the golden light of the Yang Lateral Lines and grounding into the earth through the Press Points.
- Simultaneously contract the entirety of the perineum, progressing from both Back Perineum Quadrants to both Lateral Transverse Perineals to both Front Perineum Quadrants.
- Pull and float the ensuing Rebound up internally with the entirety of your Deep Core Yin Lines—from the perineum up all the horizontal diaphragms of the inner tube of your central energy channel, while still posting all the feet Press Points and tail into the earth an energetic body length away from you.

It is extremely important to keep elongating all four sides of your body evenly. Notice which Lines your habitual posture uses and which it ignores. As stated earlier, very often the Front line is dominant, and we are oblivious to the full breadth of the Lateral Line. If this is the case for you, the following order of sequence will help. This is also the same order of progression as the Twelve Meridian Cycle, which starts at 7am with the Stomach Line.

- First run the Front Lines from your head to their extended presence through the Big Ball Press Points to their Push-away Points in the earth or space.
- Similarly, ground the Back Line into place.
- Finally, engage the Lateral Lines by wrapping from the rooted Heels to the rooted Big Balls: drawing all along the heel-foot from its posting in

the Heel; to the blade of the foot; to 5th and 4th toes; to posting in the Small Ball; to the 3rd, 2nd, and big toes of the toe-foot; and finally posting in the Big Ball.

- In this sweep from back to front, you are more likely to encompass the full breadth of the connective tissue of each Lateral Line from its furthest back edge at the buttock cheek all the way to the front of the hip bone (gluteus maximus, gluteus medius and tensor fascia lata) and feel the release down your outer thigh, which otherwise often suffers from the shortening and painful contraction of its wide ilio-tibial band, a common and debilitating occurrence both in athletes and in people who sit a lot.

The more you are able to engage the entire yang-yin connective tissue and chi meridian system, along with its corresponding Press Points and Perineum Sectors, the more you will be able to gain control of the steering mechanism of your perineum and effectively create Somatic WAves™ that strengthen your energy, muscles and inner organs as well as intensify your sexual response.

Make sure that you notice small advances as you go along and, once you gain significant improvement, remember to continue your Perineum Power asanas! The Wand* is useful to help you gain somatic awareness and to keep refining it, but throughout the day remember that you can activate and bring awareness to the components of the full asana of each Line without it.

As with any muscle, these muscles will weaken if neglected. Use ideokinesis while going about your day to keep them bouncy and vital. Maintain their tone and training to keep your perpetual "fountain of youth" pumping!

SOMATIC WAVE™ YOGA

Further application of these Perineum Power principles to movement in general, as well as to the execution of yoga postures, can be found in my upcoming book, *Surfing the Somatic WAve™ ~ Moving from the Inside Out*, which explores:

- steering specific movements with the perineum
- floating into yoga poses in "magical" ways that are appropriate to your evolving body at each moment in time

- moving from the inner core rather than the outer layer of the musculo-skeletal system
- creating safety and healing for joints
- elongating rather than stretching
- balancing Yang and Yin Lines to create physical tensegrity, stability and self-supported equipoise
- accessing challenging yoga poses through the realm of felt-sense energy and visualization

17
ORGASM AND HEALTH

Sexual ecstasy and health have an inherent connection, and orgasmic bliss is a pleasant medicine to take for your constitution! According to Dr. Christiane Northrup, author of *Women's Bodies, Women's Wisdom* (2009), their connection is scientifically proven.

Orgasm has many benefits. The 8,000 nerves in the clitoris send a direct message to the brain. During orgasm, the endothelial lining of blood vessels manufactures nitric oxide, which boosts the production of dopamine, serotonin and beta endorphin—the neurotransmitters that create euphoria and are often sought by women through Prozac!

> "Self-help and therapy are nice, but they don't accomplish a chemical shift."
>
> *Mama Gena*

In order to create this chemical shift on your own, Mama Gena's School of Womanly Arts advocates reclaiming being turned on, ". . . an experience women have been taught to avoid for the last 5,000 years. Yet the erotic is where a woman's confidence lives, where her power is sourced, where she connects to her deepest feelings and longings" (Thomashauer, 2016, p. 19).

What brings out the sensual woman in you? What longing makes your heart soar? Make love with that to empower your deep soulful self and enhance your health.

INTENSIFIED ORGASM

Opposing Force:

Intensify your pleasure with the Opposing Force that you have been developing. By combining the 'pull in' and 'pull out' directions simultaneously, you can create this chemical shift naturally, either with or without your Perineum Magic Wand. While the Press Points push out to root deeply, the combined actions of sucking with the mouth on the exhale (see Chapter 11, The Deep Core), hugging the Wand* inward and up with the yoni, pulling up with the arches of the feet and drawing the clitoris upward all stimulate the upward movement of full-body orgasm.

Simply practicing Somatic WAve™ throughout the day for postural reasons enhances the ease of orgasm because it preps the body in the use of Opposing Force and Rebound and primes it to create an upward WAve™ through the diaphragms.

Fantasy:

If you fantasize, be mindful of who or what you fantasize about in order to keep your auric field clean as well as to respect the sovereign field of others. As you may have already noticed, thought forms have a real effect in this dimension.

Flower and Fruit:

Human bodies are created to allow for physical reproduction, just like everything else that is alive on this earth. There is no derogatory word for sex in the Hawaiian language, unlike in English. In traditional Hawaiian hula *kaona* (double meaning), the female yoni is often referred to as *pua* (a flower). Feel this purity in the following metaphor.

- Feel the beautiful outer petals of your flower move as you breathe in the essence of the Earth, attracting a pollinator with your scent.
- Just as Mother Nature makes a flower beautiful to attract pollination, she makes the fruit delicious for dispersal of the pit and seed. Inside of you is the fruit that this flower has created, surrounding your juicy sexual organs.
- As the sides of your perineum draw in to pull against the Wand* or a penis, build an Opposing Force by pushing out with all the Yang Lines of your feet and tail.
- Feel the pressure build, until the Rebound cracks the pit and releases your juiciness.

ENERGY OF COLOUR

Our energy and physical bodies are not only affected by thoughts and feelings, but also by the energetic vibrations of sound and colour. Their effects on all our chakras, as well as on the major hormonal glands that they correspond to, have been studied and applied to self-evolution for thousands of years.

Take advantage of the great value of consciously running energy in your chakras and the fact that energy goes wherever your attention takes it. Increased energy draws an increased flow of stem cells and blood to wherever your attention flows.

The power of visualization to transform the physical, emotional, noetic and psychic bodies is nowhere more convincing than in the simplicity of chakra meditation. Without needing to know exactly what the darkness refers to or even "see" it, you can transform the expression of your soul in this lifetime by directing the vibration of clear colour and sound into these energy vortices.

Chakras are located at the same site as the Deep Core diaphragms that lift slow, long wave lengths to the frequency of faster, shorter wave lengths. You may find that the following visualization of colour and light will enhance your sexual response, with or without a Wand*.

- As you inhale through your feet and pelvic floor, imagine that you are drawing the silver Earth energy up into your body and grounding into the earth with your exhalations.
- As the silver energy reaches your perineum, see it illuminating the clear, cherry-red orb of your first chakra as it breathes.
- Red is a strong primal, sexual colour. Make sure that the red you visualize is a bright central shade of red (e.g., red light district). This red is the colour of physical vitality.
- Visualize a clear orange light breathing in your second chakra, at the point where your womb joins your cervix. This is the colour that inspires sensuality, feelings, emotions and creativity.
- Feel/imagine your feet arches pulsing and pulling upward along with the perineum as you breathe. Make sure to keep the Press Points of your feet grounded, however.

- Just as we were imagining in Chapter 8, pulling the muscles of the vagina up in three stages (like going up three floors on an elevator), pull the red light of the first chakra up to the orange light of the second chakra with three sips of breath.

- Simultaneously, pulse the arches of the feet upward to pull up the Earth energy and resist by pushing yang energy out with the feet Press Points.

- If you are not holding the Wand* at this time, also pulse your hands as if you are sucking up through the center of your palms while the fingers draw closer together. In Taoist Healing Love practices this is called Palm Sole Genital Breathing (Chia & Chia, 1986).

- Hold the energy in your second chakra. (If you want to cultivate the energy further, also spiral your ovaries with it; then draw it up to your kidneys and spiral them with silver light.)

- As your feet press down, visualize the energy being drawn up to join your belly to your heart, and your heart to your head.

- Feel a physical sensation of love and gratitude rising through you and bursting out of you to flow all around you, completely surrounding you in a grounded sphere of light and ecstasy.

18
THE SPIRITUAL DIMENSION OF PERINEUM POWER

THE NOW

According to many spiritual teachers, being in the Now is the secret to the art of living. The Now does not age, or know time. The more you can connect with the infinite spirit that was present, pure and innocent in you as an infant and still resides in your inner child, the more you will experience the Fountain of Youth.

Life is a mystery that continually changes and the best we can do is be in the Now in order to flow with it rather than against it. The gift of the Now is to be the infinite eternal spirit, surfing the cresting wave of time into a new life at each moment.

The awareness of our inner self, which we refine in Perineum Power, not only helps us surf the WAve™ but also enables us to be in the Now in order to sense the subtle sensations of contraction or expansive warmth with which our gut and heart are continually messaging us somatically to help us navigate through life. We develop the sensitivity to notice when and what our body is communicating to us, in order to bring us back in alignment with the infinite perfection of Now instead of following out-dated neural pathways of automatic response. It is all part of the process of waking up; we recognize that our individuality functions better when we become One with our Self in each moment.

However, in the expanded state of consciousness that we experience in our toroidal energy sphere in this practice, we also open up to our universality and the Cosmic essence of which we are a part. We grow in the awareness that we are One with the Oneness that surrounds us.

ONENESS

Each torus is a physical manifestation of the unified order of the Universe that philosophers and quantum physicists such as David Bohm called the "implicate order" and which is now commonly referred to as the "Unified Field". The New Ager calls this underlying order "Spirit" and the indigenous person says "Great Spirit", whereas the classically religious person calls this "God" or "Higher Power", but the notion of connected wholeness is all the same. According to Bohm, what we see as separate in our outside world is not separate at the quantum level.

Many psychologists believe that the root of our problems in the world today is the loss of connection. This illusion of separateness from one another, as well as a loss of connection to all parts of our self, also causes physical illness. The antidote is to understand and remember that we are One with the Oneness that surrounds us. We are One with the Universe and, therefore, we are One with each other.

Because of Oneness, connecting with the implicate order of the Universe also translates into a state of order in personal consciousness that leads to a sense of unity, peace and fulfillment. In the stillness of mind available in pure consciousness, inspiration and purpose reveal themselves on a personal level and help each individual to live a life of worth as co-creator of our shared quantum reality.

When a *physical feeling* such as love, joy or bliss accompanies this awareness, it is a true meeting of the sensing Earth Mother with the Universal Consciousnness of Spirit within us. Orgasm is a moment that brings us the possibility of experiencing the union of body and Light.

EN-LIGHT-EN

In the breathing practice of Perineum Power, we breathe in the gold and silver lights of yang and yin. Can you make a small shift to recognize that this is the Light of awareness, the Light of consciousness—the glow of light that is visible in a dark room around people who meditate a lot, the light that can be picked up by Kirilian photography?

With the Stage One Beach Ball Breath, we breathe from the light of the cosmic field all around us and condense it in the lower tan tien of our core. With Stage Two, we exhale this light down and up through our physical and energetic systems, pressing into the Field with our Press Points. With Stage Three, we hold that light at its Push-away Point, yet relax our bodies to expand and renew them with the WAve™ that Rebounds through our limbs and central energy channel, aligning and energizing our chakras, connecting our lower tan tien in the pelvis with the middle tan tien in the heart and the upper tan tien in the head, before returning into the cosmic field . . . and the cycle repeats, expanding us more and more each time into the Oneness of the Universal Energy Field, into the Oneness that you may call God, Spirit or the implicate order.

AWARENESS

Any "practice" develops through awareness. It is said that each moment of awareness is a moment of self-realization that touches our enlightenment (Chopra, 2020).

The practice of continual grounding that is intrinsic to the Perineum Power method grounds us in present moment awareness. The present moment is the only place where it is possible to *split awareness* in several directions in order to *simultaneously*:

- keep ideokinetic energy moving beyond the Press Points of the feet into the crystalline energy grid of the Earth Mother
- cleanse our out-of-body chakras* below our feet as this energy Rebounds en route to our physical body
- sense the transformational elongation of both the Yang and Yin Lines of our soma as we activate the perineum and successive diaphragms of the inner core
- cleanse and activate the in-body chakras of our central energy channel as the energy moves through our physical body and continues into the torus
- connect with the light grid of the Universal Energy Field in the toroidal sphere beyond our head and hands

- cleanse the out-of-body chakras* above our head
- be within a perpetual fountain of renewal.

* The five out-of-body chakras both below our feet and above our head draw the shared energies of the human collective and the Universe into our personal vortices of potentiality, possibility, probability and then into our body.

LOVE

Bringing awareness to *feel* this Oneness with our self, with our lover and with the Universe is a great gift that our sexuality offers to our physical, psychological and spiritual well-being. Make love with yourself, with the ocean, with the sun, with your beloved.

Grow in the Light and Love of this awareness, which is beyond ideologies and religions, yet embraces them all. Connecting with the unconditional love of Source is not the domain of any particular religion or spiritual belief.

> "Love is the connective tissue of the universe, the stuff of which we are made, the experience of being whole."
>
> *Barbara Ann Brennan*

COSMIC BODY

Sex as a spiritual dimension may seem like an alien combination of opposites to some who have been shamed by ideologies or wounded by the unconscious behaviour of people around them. May all women—and all men—be free of the denial and dis-integration of this precious life force!

> "As is the human body, so is the cosmic body."
>
> *The Upanishads*

Connecting the divine sacred powers of our human body to the cosmic body can be profound and healing. Because the Yang and Yin Lines are part of the bigger energy system that surrounds the planet Earth, when two partners who are making love visualize their yang and yin energies uniting and breathing with the toroidal energy field, their sexual experience can make their relationship more intimate and far-reaching.

Union in the toroidal field can also be a solo cultivation practice, wherein the individual becomes intimate with the Earth and the Cosmos. With the visualization of yang light flowing from the "sun beyond the sun" down the outer channels, meeting the yin energy of the Earth Mother rising up the deep inner core, it is possible to be One with All That Is in an intense experience of bliss.

TAOISM

In the Taoist Healing Love practice, one imagines the yin and yang forces as goddess and god coupling above the head and orgasming in the meeting of their energies. Their ecstatic bliss is then brought into the body, circulated through the macrocosmic orbit and condensed and stored in the energy bank of the lower tan tien.

This Taoist practice is thousands of years old. Valley orgasm (a state of prolonged whole-body orgasm when the yin and yang energies come into balance, transforming sex essence into spirit) is developed to deepen the experience of love. The sexual fluids are considered to be powerful elixers that are not to be squandered recklessly. In this practice, a man retains his seminal fluids in order to keep the content of life-giving sperm for spiritual advancement (Chia & Winn, 1984).

If you would like to explore this spiritual dimension further, I highly recommend any of the many books on Healing Love chi kung written by Grandmaster Mantak Chia or Minke De Vos, as well as those that I have already cited and listed in References.

YONI PUJA

There is a secret Hindu ritual still practiced today that also venerates the female sexual fluids. The supplicant bathes a yoni with libations and then ingests them, to ask the Divine Feminine for what he or she needs. The yoni can be a stone carving or, in some sects, the body of an actual woman—the older the yogini, the greater are her "superpowers" (Thomashauer, 2016). This is a wonderful affirmation of my original premise in Chapter 1— that our sexual energy can be cultivated and honoured, no matter what stage of life we are in as women.

19
FEELINGS

The way we feel emotionally effects a change
in our DNA and inner alchemy.

Intention and emotion are the yang and yin of manifestation. Exhaling love and gratitude into the world through the core of our being magnetizes a cascade of Grace that fills our inhales and fulfills our intentions.

Throughout this book, physical strengthening of the perineum with somatic awareness and intention has created waves in the sea of energy that enabled lungs to maximize their breathing capacity and chi meridians to infuse organs and glands with greater energy and health. Urinary, digestive, reproductive and sexual systems can now work more coherently. The connective tissues that support organs and skeleton have been strengthened and aligned within a universal blueprint of intrinsic order.

You have also learned that it is important to be aware of *emotional feelings* with your sensing soma. Otherwise, the perineum can stay fixed in a negative holding position if you are stressed, afraid, "stuck in your head" or shamed. Even the word "pudenda", a term for external female genitals still used today, is originally a Latin word meaning "to be ashamed of." How many hundreds and thousands of years have women and the female principle lived under this offensive judgment and imprecation? This attitude of abuse and exploitation is also suffered by Mother Earth.

Honouring the female principle and your own perineum can bring healing to the effects of cultural abuse passed down from many previous generations in the collective unconscious, the impact of which you may not even be aware of until you feel it arise from your subconscious during your practice. Realize that a lack of self-honouring can cause either a shaming sexual repression or a backlash of unbalanced promiscuity that is just as lacking in self-esteem. These conflicting reactions to previous generations can bounce back and forth until emotional balance is found, here at the head of your ancestral line.

FEELINGS AFFECT DNA

The new research on epigenetics has taught us that the way we feel and think about ourselves can cause changes at the level of our DNA molecules.

The DNA in every cell of your body is responding to the *feelings* of your thoughts and words. It is not the thought itself that is powerful, nor is it the action; rather, it is the magnetic field that is generated by your *feeling* body while thinking or doing. In the meditative space between thoughts, you can contact the pure consciousness of Self, where your feeling body can be refreshed in a hormonal cascade that opens you to the highest level of Self-regulation.

Bathing your female organs in a sensation of love and gratitude right now and whenever you bring attention to this area throughout the day will reclaim their health and integrity. Honouring your sexuality will also magnetize the same energy in the people and circumstances that you attract.

THE SCIENCE OF MIRACLES

> "Not all knowledge is taught in one school."
>
> *Hawaiian proverb*

I gained appreciation of the power of the feeling body as a student and dancer in a traditional hula *halau* (school) in Kauai over the past twenty years. Any dance that is an expression of the soul is powerful and mesmerizing. By embodying the intention of a *sacred* hula dance emotionally, the dancer is able not only to uplift herself but also to magnetize a higher transformative state of consciousness in the audience.

The ancients understood that the dancer needs to ground to become one with Mother Earth, move hips and breath to increase *mana* (energy) and communicate the intention of the dance through movements fueled with true emotion in order to connect with the Universal Creative Force. This was the science of miracles. Prayers without breath, energy and emotion did not travel very far in comparison; hence, the word *haole* (without breath) was applied to Westerners arriving on the islands.

Kanaloa (enlightenment) was not just a spiritual attainment but an advanced and unified state of being of all the physical, emotional, mental and spiritual selves. The ancients recognized the need to stay grounded, even while experiencing the intensity of emotion and the magnified energy of higher dimensional frequencies, in order to attain mastery. Otherwise, the dancer could be transported too far and lose her place in the dance.

THE DANCE OF LIFE

It is the same in the dance of life, if we are carried away and lose awareness and grounding.

Being in touch with the infinite within oneself, while staying grounded, somatically aware and emotionally present, gives confidence and direction in this dance of life.

> "Life is the dancer. You are the dance."
>
> *Oprah*

Fortunately, in Western culture as well, somatic awareness is increasingly recognized for its connection with, and profound influence on, our life essence. With a *physical sensation* of love and gratitude fueling the focus of your vision and conscious intention, you can participate more in the immense power of the Universe, in a manner that thought, words or action alone cannot do. Your perineum supports this potential creative power, which previously was either hidden from most women or seldom appreciated.

INNER ALCHEMY

The ancients in every part of the world practiced a secret internal alchemy that energized the body with the perineum, magnetized the central column, connected with the Higher Self and then brought this energy back down and inside in order to become integrated and whole. In India it was called tantra, in China chi kung, in Europe wicca, in Hawaii ho'oipoipo (James, 1993). These practices increased personal energy, spiritual advancement and the ability to manifest intention.

Sometimes the secrets were cloaked due to fear of misuse or misunderstanding. However, karma dispenses its own rewards or retribution. The secrets also were guarded because they gave power to those who had the knowledge, but globally the time of secrecy is now over. Women and men around the world are moving toward the dawning of global unity and understanding, and they are sharing in Oneness. If you have been attracted to this book, you are one of them.

In the modern world, inner alchemy is present in the theories of psychiatrist Carl Jung. He noticed ancient alchemical symbols mysteriously showing up in the dreams of patients and concluded that alchemy is a universal process in the awakening of illumination and inner liberation—it is not about transmuting base metals into gold. Inner alchemy creates a union of spirit and matter and the Oneness of all beings.

> "*Aurum Nostrum Non Est Aurum Vulgi:*
>
> Our gold is not common gold."
>
> *ancient Alchemist saying*

Please take a moment to recognize the gift of inner alchemy that your Perineum Power journey can give you to unify and transform your life. Take a complete breath, sensing the new aliveness in your perineum as you breathe. Feel the vastness of breath and energy moving into you, through you and out of you to join in the perpetual motion of the Universe.

See your wholeness, potential and beauty. Let these qualities fill you with a new sense of awe, gratitude and love, from the grounding of your feet in Mother Earth to the top of your head.

Be aware that the sensing and feeling muscles, organs and glands of your pelvis can now participate not only in the creation of another life, but also in the creation of your new life in concert with the Infinite.

As you fill with inner light and bliss, become the window that opens between the finite and the Infinite, giving birth to new possibilities!

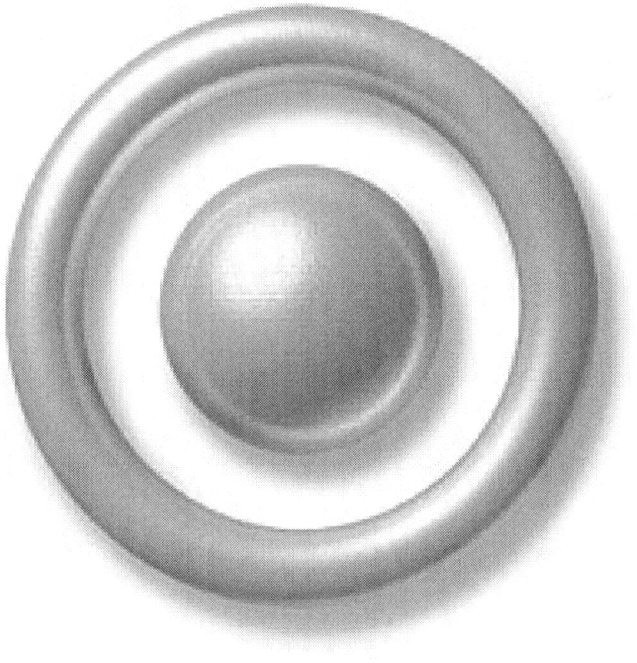

Fig. 22 Alchemy Symbol of Gold for Meditation

If you have found this book beneficial or enlightening, I invite you to:

- share a review on Amazon to let other readers know what benefits can be experienced with *Perineum Power for Women.*
- join my mailing list <PerineumPower@InnerMoves.com> so that you can be notified regarding future workshops, retreats and publications such as: *Surfing the Somatic WAve™ ~ Moving From the Inside Out.*

TESTIMONIALS FROM STUDENTS

The following testimonials were offered by students after either a private session or a group workshop. Participants were eager to send me their comments so that I would continue this work. For privacy reasons, they asked me to withhold their names or initials.

"I absolutely LOVED our session. You shared so much information with me, which was very inspiring and left me hungry for more. I especially loved engaging in the process using the beautiful tool you created for women."

"Because I have had negative experiences related to sex and sexual relationships, the sexual parts of my body can be tense. This work heals and helps to release the tension and transform it into strength and sensation."

"The lessons were given with a spirit of delicacy, privacy and step-by-step directions to avoid feelings of awkwardness."

"I feel such integration between inner and outer bodies. I feel more connected to myself."

"The sessions were very healing and inspiring. I was able to connect with the tremendous power of the perineum and entire inner energy channel, and to feel this connection ongoing whenever I bring awareness to it."

"I feel more in touch with my innards, kidneys, lungs, ovaries."

"I use the Wand* regularly and am very grateful. Thank you for creating it. It has replaced the jade egg for me. So lovely!"

"I can articulate the perineum quadrants better."

"It supports me in how I carry myself in movement, breathing and meditation."

"As I age and my outer body becomes perhaps less strong and flexible or deals with injuries, I can see that even if I become limited in my movement, I will be able to work my body from the inside out."

"It inspires me to continue to access and explore what my body is and can be."

"I felt at peace after each session."

"The workshop was done in a safe and sensitive way… relaxing and opening with trust."

"My body had a complete and total awareness as one, inside and out."

"Energy lines from the feet to the top of the head were no longer stopping and starting around the pelvis or lower back area."

"My internal pelvic/perineum muscles became stronger very quickly."

"My large intestine elimination system became normal and healthy within 24 hours."

"This was a remarkable experience—a balanced feeling of joy and restful peace combined and lasted for days. It became possible to re-activate these feelings by concentrating on the perineum and with breathing exercises."

"I truly wish all could experience this in their own way."

REFERENCES

Batson, G. (2013). Exercise-induced central fatigue: a review of the literature with implications for dance science research. *Journal of Dance Medicine & Science, 17*(2), 53–62. doi:10.12678/1089-313X.17.2.53, PMID 23759479

Bartkow, D. (2012). Embodiment of light and love – Chakra meditation. https://www.innermoves.com/meditation

Berzuk, K. (2002). *I laughed so hard I peed my pants!* Incontinence & Pelvic Pain Clinic.

Chevalier, G., Sinatra, S. T., Oschman, J. L., Sokal, K., & Sokal, P. (2012). Earthing: health implications of reconnecting the human body to the Earth's surface electrons. *Journal of Environmental and Public Health, 2012*, 291541. doi.org/10.1155/2012/291541

Chia, M. (2004). *Cosmic inner smile, smiling heals the body.* Universal Tao Publications.

Chia, M. (2016). Introduction to non Taoist inner alchemy levels of immortality. Retrieved from https://www.mantakchia.com/immortal-inner-alchemy-teaching-master-mantak-chia/

Chia, M. & Chia, M. (1986). *Cultivating female sexual energy.* Healing Tao Books.

Chia, M. & Winn, M. (1984). *Taoist secrets of love, cultivating male sexual energy.* Aurora Press.

Chopra, D. (2020). *Hope in uncertain times – 21-Day meditation experience. (Day 21).* https://www.chopracentermeditation.com/experience

De Vos, M. (2016). *Tao tantric arts for women.* Inner Traditions.

Fogel, A. (2010, July 7). *Slow movement with awareness: Better than exercise?* Retrieved from https://www.psychologytoday.com/ca/blog/body-sense/201007/slow-movement-awareness-better-exercise

Gach, M. (2020). Online acupressure trainings. https://www.acupressurecircle.com

Hanna, T. (1979). *The body of life.* Alfred A. Knopf.

Hawkins, D. R. (2002). *Power VS. force: The hidden determinants of human behaviour.* Hay House.

James, T. & James, A. (1993). *Lost secrets of ancient Hawaiian huna.* Ka Ha O Hawaii Foundation.

Jensen, L. T., & Jensen, N. M. (2005). *Daughters of Haumea.* Pueo Press.

Kaparo, R. (2001). *Yoga mastery and somatic meditations course reader.*

Keleman, S. (1985). *Emotional anatomy.* Center Press.

Mutual Publishing. (2003). *Hula ~ Hawaiian proverbs and inspirational quotes.*

Myers, R. W. (2001). *Anatomy trains – Myofascial meridians for manual and movement therapists.* Churchill Livingstone Elsevier.

Myers, R. W. (2009). *Anatomy trains – Myofascial meridians for manual and movement therapists* (2nd ed.). Churchill Livingstone Elsevier.

Nia, (2020). https://nianow.com/nia-5-stages.

Northrup, C. (2009). *Women's bodies, women's wisdom: The complete guide to women's health and wellbeing.* Piatkus Publishing.

Oschman, J., Streeter, T. W. J. A., Soh, K. S., Jones, J., Langevin, H. M., & Hp Mae Wan. (2016). Slide 41-638 [diagram of polygonal structure of an acupoint]. https://www.slideshare.net/thorntonstreeter/primo-vascularmeridian-system-2016

Rolf, I. P. (1987). *Rolfing: The integration of human structures.* Harper Collins.

Scaravelli, V. (1991). *Awakening the spine.* Harper Collins.

Thie, J. (1994). *Touch for health* (revised ed.). DeVorss Publications.

Thomashauer, R. (2016). *Pussy, a reclamation.* Hay House, Inc.

Yung, K. T. (2004). A birdcage model of the Chinese meridian system: Part 1. A channel as a transmission line. Am J Chin Med. 2004; 32: 815- 828. [*Journal of Acupuncture and Meridian Studies,* (Dec. 2013). *6*(6), 331-338] https://doi.org/10.1016/j.jams.2013.10.001

ABOUT THE AUTHOR

Dhyana Bartkow, MA, BEd, ARCT and Black Belt is the founder of Inner Moves Wellness Center on the Sunshine Coast of British Columbia, Canada. As well as receiving clients for classes, bodywork and personal retreats at the studio location in Gibsons, she also hosts workshops and conscious community gatherings at Crystal Creek Nature Retreat, the forest facility on Mount Elphinstone.

A certified Black Belt Nia instructor and a traditional Hawaiian Hula, yoga and meditation teacher, Dhyana is also a *lomilomi* (Hawaiian shamanic bodywork) and acupressure practitioner, as well as an aura healer.

Dhyana has taught in Canada, Hawaii and Mexico. As a pioneeer in holistic fitness arts who created the first mind-body-spirit fitness program in Vancouver, she was contracted to create transformational movement and meditation experiences for hundreds of participants at Peak Potentials personal growth camps.

Her productions include a 70-minute instructional movement DVD, filmed on Kauai, called "Inner Moves in Hawaii" and two meditation CDs, "Embodiment of Light and Love Chakra Meditation" and "Elemental Meditations of the Heart," which are available on her website, www.InnerMoves.com.

Dhyana is the creator of the revolutionary movement and energy work technique, Somatic WAve™, of which Perineum Power is a central component. She has also written the manual *Surfing the Somatic WAve™ ~ Moving from the Inside Out.* In this method, balanced movement and healing is initiated from energy channels and core diaphragms rather than by external muscles and bones. This technique is appropriate for both the beginner and the more advanced yoga student who is looking for intrinsic routes to more complex poses; it also serves as a healing method for the injured.

Her background as an educator and information researcher, combined with her personal quest to heal from three severe skeletal injuries, motivated her extensive research in this field of wellness. Along with self-enquiry, it has given her a deep understanding of the human body and the energy body. This personal journey brings compassion to her training and teaching experience, inspiring others with faith in the possibility to heal and thrive.

"As a conference producer,
I give Dhyana a 5-star rating.
She provides a rare combination of creativity
and practicality that allows people to
discover and express their essence."

Harv Eker, Peak Potentials

Dhyana may be contacted at:
Inner Moves Wellness Center, www.InnerMoves.com
Gibsons BC Canada
Info@InnerMoves.com

Manufactured by Amazon.ca
Bolton, ON

33932992R00077